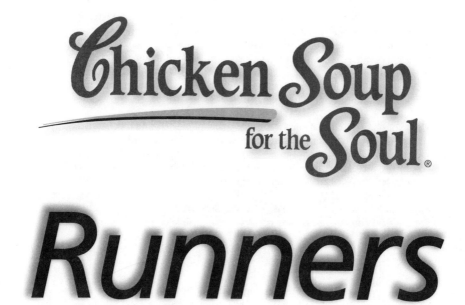

Runners

D0071749

Chicken Soup for the Soul: Runners
101 Inspirational Stories of Energy, Endurance, and Endorphins
by Jack Canfield, Mark Victor Hansen, Amy Newmark,
and Ultramarathoner Dean Karnazes
Published by Chicken Soup for the Soul Publishing, LLC   www.chickensoup.com

The publisher gratefully acknowledges the many publishers and individuals who
granted Chicken Soup for the Soul permission to reprint the cited material.

*Cover photo provided courtesy The North Face. Back cover photo provided courtesy True
Alliance. Interior photo provided courtesy of Caio Guatelli.*

Cover and Interior Design & Layout by Pneuma Books, LLC
For more info on Pneuma Books, visit www.pneumabooks.com

Distributed to the booktrade by Simon & Schuster. SAN: 200-2442

Publisher's Cataloging-in-Publication Data
(Prepared by The Donohue Group)

Chicken soup for the soul : runners : 101 inspirational stories of energy,
  endurance, and endorphins / [compiled by] Jack Canfield ... [et al.].

    p. ; cm.

  ISBN: 978-1-935096-49-8

1. Runners (Sports)--United States--Anecdotes. 2. Runners (Sports)--United States-
-Literary collections. 3. Running--Anecdotes. 4. Running--Literary collections. 5.
Physical fitness--Anecdotes. 6. Physical fitness--Literary collections. I. Canfield,
Jack, 1944- II. Title: Runners

PN6071.R7 C45 2010
810.8/02/0357   2010924960

PRINTED IN THE UNITED STATES OF AMERICA
on acid∞free paper
17 16 15 14 13 12 11 10   01 02 03 04 05 06 07 08

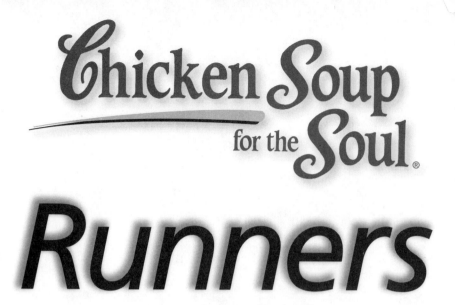

Chicken Soup for the Soul
Runners

101 Inspirational Stories of
Energy, Endurance, and
Endorphins

Jack Canfield
Mark Victor Hansen
Amy Newmark
and Ultramarathoner
Dean Karnazes

Chicken Soup for the Soul Publishing, LLC
Cos Cob, CT

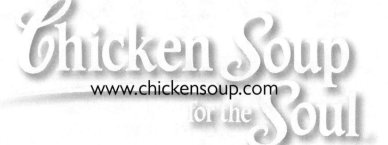

www.chickensoup.com

Contents

❶

~Starting Out~

❷

~Running Therapy~

❸

~Camaraderie~

❹

~Comebacks~

❺

~Everyday Adventures~

❻

~Family Ties~

❼

~A Step at a Time~

❽

~Fortitude~

❾

~Interesting Places~

⑩
~Moving on to Triathlons~

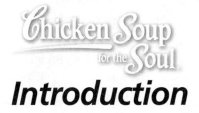

Introduction

When all else fails, start running.
~Dean Karnazes

I got sick of living the life that everybody told me I *should* be living, so one day I decided to start living life on my own terms. Frustrated with my job, I found myself in a bar on the eve of my 30th birthday preparing to drink the night away. Instead, I walked out at 11:00 PM, and just started running... and running and running. I hadn't run in the past decade, and that fateful evening I ran thirty miles non-stop straight through the night. That single inspired (okay, some may say crazy) act forever changed the course of my life.

Ironically, it was my boss who provided the impetus for this departure. Perhaps a bit ahead of her time, she took particular interest in her employees' overall satisfaction instead of only monitoring workplace performance. She gave each of us a copy of *Chicken Soup for the Soul* and encouraged us to read a story or two. I was intrigued. This was not your typical business-related book!

Many of my colleagues would hit the bars after a tough day at work. My boss would instead curl up and read some inspirational anecdotes in her book. Me, I started running as a way to decompress.

But I also started reading. Interestingly enough, I found many similarities between the two; *Chicken Soup for the Soul* and running both nourished my inner spirit. They complemented each other perfectly!

The *Chicken Soup for the Soul* series is a collection of uplifting and energizing short stories. The concept is simple, yet powerful. Running, too, is simple, yet powerful. By its very nature, running is a moving experience, both literally and figuratively!

As any athlete can attest, running conditions the body. The stories I started reading daily in *Chicken Soup for the Soul* were perfect cross-training for the soul. When I was feeling lazy or unmotivated, reading a stirring and heartwarming story reinvigorated my sense of passion and commitment, and off I'd go on a run!

Apparently, I'm not the only one who finds this to be the case. Since its initial release back in 1993, the *Chicken Soup for the Soul* series has sold more than 500 million copies worldwide, making it one of the bestselling books of all time. And there are now more than 200 titles in circulation. Clearly, we humans are social animals and reading about others overcoming incredible adversity and living life to its fullest empowers us to do the same. When I learned about this new *Chicken Soup for the Soul* title dedicated entirely to runners, I was supremely honored when asked to be a part it!

Since walking out of that bar on the eve of my 30th birthday and running off into the night, my life has been completely transformed. I decided to make my passion for running my vocation. I had no idea how I was going to do this, but I just figured if I followed my heart and did what I loved, I could somehow make a go of it. If nothing else, I'd certainly be a lot happier than if I continued going to work every day in a job I didn't enjoy.

Of course, it was a terrifying leap of faith to trust my instincts. I would be giving up the plush corner office, the corporate perks, healthcare coverage, the 401K matching program, etc… How would I live without these things?

I'll never forget telling my wife, Julie, about my decision to leave the corporate world. Her response to me was revealing. "Well," she said, "I was wondering how long it would take you." With that kind of support and encouragement, there was no turning back!

It's been a wild run ever since. I've been able to travel the globe, often taking Julie and our two great kids along for the ride. We've seen some of the most exotic places on Earth, and met some of the most remarkable people along the way. I've participated in hundreds of marathons and ultramarathons in just about every imaginable setting, from the blazing summertime heat of Death Valley to the frigid cold of the South Pole. Life's become an amazing adventure, and it just keeps getting better every day!

I've come to believe that enthusiasm flows from doing what you're passionate about. It's so exciting to see people learn about my story and watch them get excited too. Never in my wildest dreams could I have imagined making *TIME* magazine's "Top 100 Most Influential People in the World" list. But there was my name, at number 27 no less! What this illustrated to me was that my message of following your heart and living life with passion and purpose resonated strongly with a lot of people.

I share my personal story with you not to be boastful, but to provide you with the conviction that you, too, can steer your life in any direction you so desire. Sometimes all it takes is that spark of inspiration to ignite a burning passion within!

Which brings me back to *Chicken Soup for the Soul: Runners*. In this book you will find a wide collection of authors, from elite Olympians to casual joggers, all with the same intention, to provide you with a ray of hope that life can indeed be a fantastic and fulfilling journey.

There's something undeniably empowering about reading stories of others who have brushed aside their fears and taken great risks to be all that they can be. To read firsthand about the trials, tribulations, hardships and setbacks others have faced is emotionally rousing. To see the grit, determination and perseverance they have displayed in pursuing their dreams is deeply stirring. These amazing stories provide, dare I say it, nourishment for the soul.

If reading this book motivates you to lace up your running shoes and head out the door, I say go with it! My hope is that *Chicken Soup for the Soul: Runners* will inspire you to be the very best that you can be, whether you run great distances, modest distances, or not at all. A life worth living is meant to be an impassioned journey, one in which we continue to explore, learn and expand our potential each and every day. I encourage you to find your edge, and then take a step beyond it. This stride into the unknown is where true discovery begins. I wish you the very best of luck on your journey!

With that said, I'm off for a run.

Catch ya down the road...
~Dean

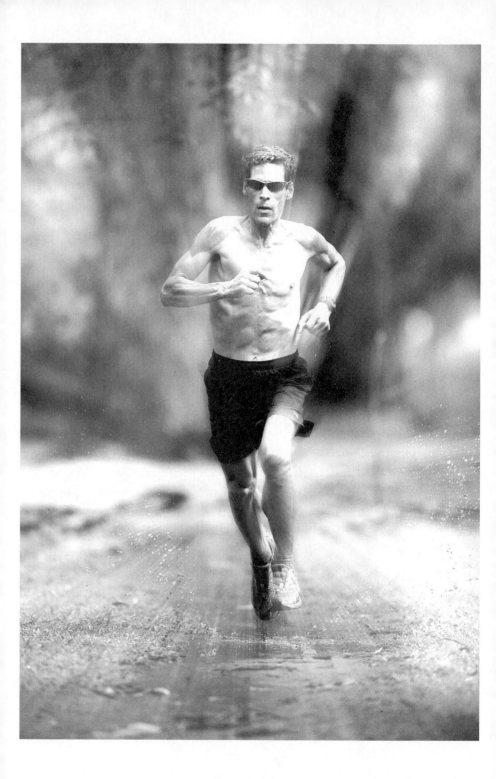

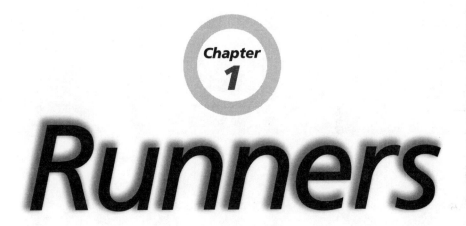

Chapter 1

Runners

Starting Out

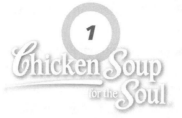

The Circle
Is the Only Geometry

I've learned that finishing a marathon isn't just an athletic achievement. It's a state of mind; a state of mind that says anything is possible.
~John Hanc

awn had just lifted the covers off a gray, drizzly Monday morning in April 1983 when my mom came to my room and, not quite literally, dragged me from bed. After a quick breakfast the whole family piled into Dad's Saab and we travelled two hours southwest to the Boston suburb of Hopkinton, where the 87th Boston Marathon would begin at noon.

In Hopkinton we hooked up with our friend Dori, a local who knew the area inside and out and guided us to three or four good cheering points along the course while Dad, running his first marathon as a numberless bandit, made the 26.2-mile eastward journey to Copley Square on foot. We reached the first viewing spot in time to see the race leaders, already far ahead of our patriarch, among whom were the legendary Bill Rodgers and Joan Benoit. The frontrunner, local boy Greg Meyer, sailed by faster than I could sprint. We were awestruck.

Our final stop was Cleveland Circle, at 25 miles. We waited and waited. At last Dad came, in what looked like a slow-motion replay of his previous stride, his massive size-14 feet landing heavily, his shoulders sagging, his weary eyes staring a thousand miles ahead. As planned, my two brothers and I broke from the curb and jogged with him over the last mile to the finish line, like three Navy cruisers flanking an aircraft carrier.

It was the coolest thing ever. Being cheered along by a seemingly endless, six-deep gauntlet of shouting spectators was like sudden fame. And although we'd never heard of Bill Rodgers or Joan Benoit until that day, our impressionable ten- to fourteen-year-old minds made instant heroes of them.

The next morning at breakfast Josh, the eldest, announced that he was going to start running, and so did I. After school we ran our dad's favorite 6-mile route on mostly dirt roads surrounding our home. Two days later, we did it again. Twenty-seven years later, I'm still running.

Only last year, however, did I get around to running the entire Boston Marathon myself. I meant to do it sooner. I tried to do it sooner. But there were problems. Always problems. In 2001 I got injured two weeks before the race. The next four years were lost to various other injuries.

At last I made it to Hopkinton healthy, but the curse followed me. My right shoe was scraped off my foot by the toe of a runner behind me just half a mile into the race. I got it back on, but my relief was short-lived. Around the 10K mark I felt a twinge in my right hamstrings, and the pain grew steadily worse thereafter. At 12 miles, with a jolt of panic, I felt the first hint of a soreness destined to become an agony in both thighs. Less than halfway and already my shock absorbers were blown!

As the pain in my thighs worsened, I began to look ahead to the 16-mile mark—where my parents, Josh, his wife, and even Dori awaited my triumphant passage—as a potential place to drop out. (Only my younger brother, Sean, was missing from the original crew; he followed my race online at home in California.) But when I spotted my personal cheering section in the crowd, my conscience was seared by a sense of obligation to honor their support and I kept running, hoping for the best and fearing the worst.

Right away I regretted my decision. Despite my best efforts at mind over matter, my pace continued to slow, until I could not run—I mean *could not run*—another step. I switched from a rigid shuffle to a herky-jerky walk just shy of the 23-mile mark. It brought amazingly little relief. I now doubted my ability to even *walk* to the finish line.

I was more miserable than I had ever been in any previous race, and believe me, that's saying something. Each step was a thousand daggers poked deeply into the tender flesh of my thighs.

On top of everything else, the air was freezing—47 degrees, to be precise—and my body produced far less heat while walking than running. I shivered like Leonardo di Caprio in the last scene of *Titanic* under the flimsy space blanket I had snatched from a First Aid station. I no longer cared at all about finishing. If a concerned onlooker had offered me a ride back to Dori's house I would have seized the offer without shame, like an emaciated desert crawler gobbling pig slop.

Offering rides was the last thing on the minds of the spectators who thickly lined the last miles of the Boston Marathon course along Commonwealth Avenue. Instead they hollered encouragement as though their lives depended on the performance of every runner. I drew special attention from the crowd because of my obvious plight, which only deepened the humiliation of my failure. *Just leave me alone!* I thought.

Then, all of a sudden, I found myself at Cleveland Circle, where my brothers and I had broken from the curb to guide our dad home so long ago, and I realized that, despite earlier doubts, this awful nightmare would eventually end. A slight diminishment of the agony in my thighs suggested that I might even be able to jog the last mile and get it over with that much faster. As I contemplated giving it a try I realized that discarding my space blanket and breaking into stride might appear rather theatrical given the amount of attention being heaped upon me. I wished I could attempt the experiment unnoticed, but that was impossible, so I sheepishly scanned the faces in the throng on the left side of the course for the inevitable reaction as I dashed the blanket to the road and began jogging.

My eyes met those of three frat-boy types in baseball caps who were among those urging me *personally* toward the finish, almost belligerent in their support. And as I seemingly responded to their urgings by giving them exactly what they demanded of me, they pumped their fists in the air, high-fived, and, through exultant laughter, shouted, "YEAH!", repeating the behaviors they had undoubtedly exhibited when the Red Sox beat the Yankees in game seven of the 2004 American League Championship Series. My pathetic little comeback seemed to have made them as happy as they had been in their entire lives. I had to laugh too.

My dad is fond of saying, "The circle is the only geometry." He means that, throughout life, we continually return to the beginning. I recalled this expression when, on the exact spot where I became a runner as a boy, I became a runner again as a nearly middle-aged man. Until that moment I was filled with disappointment over having failed to run as fast as I wanted to run, not just in this marathon but throughout my running life. But in that moment I was reminded of what a blessing it is to be able to run at all, and what a wonderful gift my dad had given me on a drizzly Monday in April 1983.

~Matt Fitzgerald

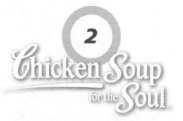

How I Found
My Running Partner

Beware of the chair!
~Author Unknown

One morning I started to sweat. Profusely. Just sitting down. I would have attributed it to hot flashes, but I knew those were years away. The accompanying pain in my left arm was what made me ask a neighbor for a ride to the emergency room.

The heart attack was minor in nature, but a major scare. Who knew that a size 2 forty-year-old who ate plenty of veggies, hated junk food, and only ate lean meats would be a candidate for heart problems? After one night of observation in the emergency room I headed home.

My doctor blamed my sedentary lifestyle for my new health problems and told me I needed to get some daily exercise. He said that because I worked at home, I lacked the need to go out, walk around an office building, walk at lunch, run for trains, and all that. I simply walked from my bedroom each morning, headed to the kitchen for coffee, and walked about 35 feet to my office. Sometimes still in my jammies.

He told me to start running. Slowly at first, maybe 50 feet, stop, walk, rest, run another 50 feet. He told me perhaps I could run each day with my husband, an accomplished headstrong runner who could do five miles a day without even breathing hard. I knew for a fact that my husband would never allow me to accompany him and slow him down, but I was ready to promise my doctor anything in order to stop the lecture.

The following day, Karen, the neighbor who had driven me to the hospital, came over to check on me. I told her I had my marching orders, or rather, my walking orders. Karen knew how much I detested exercising and laughed at my predicament.

Then she said, "I have an idea! Roxy loves to go to the park!" Roxy was her nine-year-old Lab, and we were crazy about each other. I frequently took her for her afternoon walks when Karen was away on business. "With my travel schedule, I can't take her as often as I'd like. Why don't you take her?"

Before I could answer, we heard some barking. Our yards were connected by a two-way gate that Roxy had mastered. As we watched her padding across the lawn and up my back stairs, we were astonished to see that Roxy had somehow managed to find her leash and bring it with her! As she pranced through the kitchen door, she proudly wagged her tail as she dropped the leash at my feet, and extended her paw in a "high five."

"How did you get her to do this?" I asked Karen. The entire episode smelled of conspiracy! Karen, however, couldn't stop laughing and swore up and down she had nothing to do with this!

I picked up the leash and headed out the front door with Roxy in tow. She led me down the block to the park where she promptly took off like a wild bronco! Up, down, around bushes and trees, other dogs, other owners, hills, dales and doggy hydrants. I couldn't even get her to slow down enough so I could take her leash off! And she seemed to know exactly what she was doing. She had this all planned! I finally begged for mercy as I sweated, gulped for air, and headed to the bubbler.

As I walked her home, Roxy was calm and kept glancing over at me with what looked like concern. She would slow down, look up, and when I nodded to say, "I'm fine, girl," she'd pick up the pace a bit.

The following day I had a deadline I was certain I wouldn't meet.

Being a freelance writer, this was my life. As I worked diligently, I heard Roxy barking out back. This was nothing unusual—Roxy loved to bark at the neighborhood squirrels and kids coming home from school. But something made me get up this time and go look.

Sure enough—here came Roxy, leash in her mouth, heading up my kitchen stairs! Same time as the day before! I was sure Karen had put her up to it this time, so figuring Karen was hiding in the bushes outside, I called her cell phone, knowing she'd pick up.

"Okay, lady, how on Earth did you train Roxy to do this?"

Karen seemed befuddled. "Huh?"

"The leash thing! She looks so cute sitting here with the leash in her mouth!" I explained.

"She's at your house? Good grief! She must have gone out the doggy door in the basement. I am at the grocery store and she was sleeping when I left!"

I just looked down at Roxy, and I knew. This was her idea. She knew how to help me. And she was doing it.

This routine went on for almost three years. Every day, rain or shine, Roxy showed up with her leash and barked at my kitchen door. I could set my clock by her: 3:00 on the dot, every day.

My doctor was thrilled and I was feeling wonderful. I actually toned up with all this running and chasing and doggy babysitting. I loved spending time with Roxy. It gave me something to look forward to each day.

Even though I wasn't officially "jogging," I was certainly doing my share of running! Maybe without form, but certainly with lots of purpose. Roxy would never let me take off her leash! She seemed to instinctively know I needed to be attached to her in order to get better! Many of our doggy dates ended up with a healthy frozen yogurt at the park, which I lovingly shared with her.

Then one morning my phone rang very early. Caller ID told me it was Karen, and my heart skipped a beat. No one calls at 6:00 with good news.

I picked up the phone and simply said, "What's wrong?"

She was crying. "Can you come over?"

I ran through the backyard in my robe and slippers, not knowing what I'd find. Karen opened her kitchen door for me.

"She's gone. I can't believe it. I tried to wake her for breakfast and she was cold. At least she died in her sleep; she didn't suffer like I thought she might. I didn't want to tell you, but she had a bad heart. It was a matter of time."

I looked at our beloved Roxy, all curled up in her warm cozy bed, peaceful and quiet—with her leash next to her, ready for our afternoon outing. I couldn't help but think that maybe we managed to keep each other alive a little longer than was meant to be.

That was almost ten years ago. I still run, but this time I have my own Lab, Sally, a gift from my husband.

It's now Sally's job to put me through my paces at the doggy park, and she does a marvelous job. Each day as we walk out the front door, Sally barks once, and wags her tail, looking at the large white urn on the bookshelf. This is where Roxy's ashes are, in loving memory. As I see Sally bark at the urn each day, I can't help but wonder, "Does she know?"

~Marie Duffoo

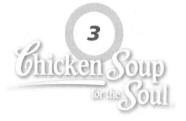

Real Runners

Life is a long lesson in humility.
~James Matthew Barrie

I t all started when I ran across a "how to" article on running in a magazine. Day one consisted of walking for 30 minutes—yes, walking. I could do that, I thought confidently. Day two added one-minute stretches of running interspersed with walking. I could do anything for a single minute, I mused. The program ever so gradually evolved into more running than walking until, at the end of eight weeks, you'd be running for 30 minutes—a couple of miles—without stopping. All you had to do was follow the plan.

That first day I called up my friend Linda and casually asked her if she'd like to go for a walk. I didn't tell her until we had already hit the trail that I was embarking on a "plan." Adding one minute of running the next day sounded reasonable to Linda, too, and she wholeheartedly signed on. We could do this. I borrowed a stopwatch, and we were on our way.

We stuck to the plan, even though those one-minute intervals seemed to last an eternity. We spent the recovery times discussing the daily events of our lives until the stopwatch beeped again, demanding another spurt of effort.

On the fourth or fifth day it rained, and we hesitated… but always one or the other of us would spur the other on. Several weeks passed, and we had completed half the program and were now running more than we were walking. We both went out and bought quality running shoes and dug up water bottles to carry with us… we were becoming real runners after all. We continued our regimen religiously, and now we chatted even during the running portion of our training. We shared our hopes, dreams, and fears, developing a deep bond while facing the physical challenges and pushing ourselves to accomplish our goal.

At the end of eight weeks we were running 30 minutes straight. It might not seem like much to a real runner, but as two previously non-athletic moms sneaking up on middle age, we were thrilled with the accomplishment. And then we did what all real runners do—we signed up for a race: a 5K just a few weeks away.

With newfound confidence from having completed our program and continuing to give each other encouragement, we anxiously pinned paper numbers to our T-shirts and then started and finished our first official race. It was an amazing high for us. We had become real runners!

A few days later we went out to run together again. Parking at a trailhead we did our pre-run stretching behind the car. Leaning against the trunk with our hands, we lengthened our legs behind us to stretch out our hamstrings—just as we'd learned from the running magazine. We were both still jazzed up from our recent triumph. Our heads were filled with images of ourselves as buff athletes, our bodies finely tuned running machines—real runners who ran in races! But it soon became apparent that our new status was not yet obvious to the general public. Our reverie and self-congratulations were interrupted when not one, but two cars slowed down and stopped, the driver of one leaning out his window. "Do you ladies need help pushing your car?" he offered generously.

~Marjorie Woodall

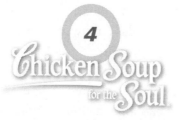

The Side Effect of Fear

The greatest stimulator of my running career was fear.
~Herb Elliott

Who in their right mind would think that terror could be good? Granted, it's mostly bad. But it can be a marvelous stimulant in the young life of an aspiring runner, even if the reason he's running is sheer terror.

I have the ignominious distinction of having been chased home by a girl nearly every day of my third-grade life. I suppose I ought to thank Laura, wherever she is, for being the catalyst for my running habit. Those who lived along Highland Street in Laconia might have remarked, "What a healthy young man! Always running!" But if they were patient, they might have perhaps seen, far in the distance, a tall young woman in a black leather jacket trotting along. And perhaps if they studied my pale face, they might have seen the telltale signs of fear: the quivering lip, the wide eyes. Perhaps they even saw me looking back over my shoulder every few steps.

I was small for my age. Hell, I was small for any age, up until the eighth grade, when I shot up six inches. But up until then I was pretty miniature. And so even after Laura tired of chasing me (I heard later that she thought I was cute, though I still believe she wanted to kill me), I stuck with my habit of running to and from school. The school district had determined that my house was just a bit too close to the middle school for me to be able to take the bus. So I would run there in the morning, and run back after school. It was the after-school runs that were harrowing.

A kid running to school simply suggests lateness, which is acceptable. Even tough kids don't want to get detention for being late all the time.

But a kid running home from school; well, there's no sugar-coating that one. He's just plain old scared. And those curious hooligans at Memorial Middle School got awfully suspicious. They must have thought, why in the hell is he running all the time? So, ironically, they began chasing me home because I was running. Talk about a self-fulfilling prophecy.

Winter was the worst. For one thing, it's harder to run in the snow. And then there's the added trouble of snowballs. The availability of snowballs meant that not only must I outrun my aggressors, but that I must keep a cushion of at least forty yards between myself and them. Also, if I cut through a backyard, it became easy to track me.

When I sprouted up to 5'10" in eighth grade, they stopped chasing me. But I kept my habit of running anyway, and naturally I joined the track team. I'd found that in my daily flights of terror from school to home, I'd built up decent stamina. Not only that, but thanks to the prevalence of stone walls in backyards around Laconia, I'd been inadvertently practicing hurdling the whole time. I ran track all through high school, specializing in hurdles. While I didn't break any records, I became captain of the track team, and prepared myself for Army Basic Training, a large part of which revolves around running. And running. And running.

Even as a teacher at a school for kids with ADHD I've found a use for my long-lived running habit. I highly recommend that you try catching a kid with ADHD who's running away from you through the forest at top speed. You won't forget it. Those kids don't tire, let me tell you. But luckily for me I've been running my whole life, and even though I'm past thirty, I know how to pace myself, and they always give in eventually. I'm all done being afraid. But the running, the running has stayed with me: The lovely, unlooked-for side effect of fear.

~Ron Kaiser, Jr.

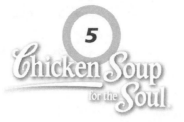

Tale of a Former Slowpoke

Little by little one walks far.
~Peruvian Proverb

"In three weeks," shouted my middle school gym teacher, "the sixth grade will begin our annual physical fitness testing. Be prepared to complete at least fifteen push-ups and a minimum of twenty sit-ups correctly, and, of course, the mile run, which must be finished within 10 minutes and 50 seconds. We will practice these three activities during gym class up until the test."

The entire P.E. class groaned in unison, and my moan was the loudest of all. I recalled the fifth grade fitness test I had taken the previous year. I had easily pulled through push-ups and crunches, but I was worst in my class when it came to running. I'm not sure what I despised most—watching the athletic kids lounge in the grass, mile completed, while I was still on my second lap, stopping to catch my breath 2 minutes into the test and hiding my face from passing runners, or feeling my legs ache and clutching the cramps in my side as I crossed the finish line, 13 minutes and 40 seconds after the test began.

In short, I was a slowpoke.

I was mortified to run the mile. For me, it meant humiliation for being the slowest in the class, as well as physical pain and too much sweat. Not to mention the fact that I would have no one to run with—all my good friends were much faster than me. I found myself worrying for the rest of the day, nervous about gym class the next morning, where we'd have to practice the timed mile.

Despite my pleas to stay home from school, I stood shivering at the school track during first period. And, as my teacher explained the run once more, I made a last-minute, desperate decision to stick with my fastest friend, the most athletic girl in the grade, for as long as I could during the run.

I didn't think much of my brash choice at first—I figured that I'd be forced to resume my normal, tortoise-like pace halfway through lap one. But as we lined up behind the starting line, a crooked crack in the pavement, I became resolute. The sharp whistle blew, and we took off. My friend, whose name was Lily, sped ahead of the entire class in three long strides. Sucking in monstrous amounts of air, I sprinted right behind her. Every time I felt the urge to stop and collapse on the dewy grass, I pushed my body a bit farther. When I finally gave in to my self-pleas and slowed to a walk, I realized that I had lasted half of a mile running directly behind Lily.

Although I walked the remaining half mile, I finished before some of my faster friends. Shocked though I was at my unexpected skill, I couldn't help but believe that it was a fluke. A one-time event. That I'd never run quickly again. So, I took action. Every night for the rest of the week, I ran up and down my street, building myself up in preparation for next week's gym class. Once I could successfully jog the entire road without pausing, I felt I was ready to dash through the mile.

My progress was slow but sure over the course of the next few months. First, I dropped behind Lily after three quarters a mile. Next, sooner to the end. Then, I finished only 10 seconds after her. By the end of the semester, I was running alongside Lily for an entire mile. My gym teachers and friends were shocked at my sudden change of pace.

When we changed P.E. groups, I became the fastest girl in my class. I was, surprisingly enough, enjoying Wednesday morning gym class—while my peers trudged sleepily outside to the track, my walk was brisk and energetic. My parents were astonished when I began jogging after school and on weekends, especially considering I'd never attempted, much less enjoyed, a sport in my life. My physical fitness test mile time earned me a spot on the coveted list duct-taped to the door of the girls' locker room, the piece of paper that told the entire school who passed the evaluation with flying colors.

As I entered seventh grade, my family was nonetheless surprised at my decision to join the middle school cross country team. To my great disappointment, our "team practices" entailed running a single lap around our miniscule track followed by several games of capture the flag. I was unfazed, however. I simply took matters into my own hands. I started training on my own time—at parks, at home, at the gym—wherever I could, until I was running daily. In addition to cross country meets, I competed in local races, increasing speed, distance, and endurance as I went. At my mother's request, I began eating about three times as much food as I did previously, considering the number of calories I burned exercising each week. I was healthy, strong, and feeling great about myself.

Towards the end of seventh grade, I took on a new venture—training for an intensive cross country camp located in rural Vermont. The camp would also include mountain biking and distance swimming as cross-training for runners. I knew that such an endeavor would be treacherous for me, a former slowpoke with very little running experience, but I made up my mind to take on the challenge.

So the training began. A spring and summer of running and exhaustion, nervousness for camp and pride for my newfound strength. And, thanks to my persistent mother, a spring and summer of intense eating and the occasional rest. The day before camp arrived at last, and amidst frantic packing, I found a sense of calm. The lingering fear of unreadiness and weakness had disappeared. I had worked hard and made an incredible transformation from slowpoke to real cross country runner. My only emotion was determination to give the week my all and do my absolute best at camp, no matter how hard it was.

The week was difficult, but rewarding—I'm proud to say that although I was far from the best runner at camp, I tried my best and definitely gained speed and endurance. I plan on continuing cross country running in eighth grade, high school and even after I graduate.

Yes, running has gotten me into shape. Far more importantly though, I've learned a ton about myself since I began the sport. I can truly do anything if I set my mind on it, even if it seems more than impossible.

Take it from a former slowpoke.

~Claire Howlett, age 13

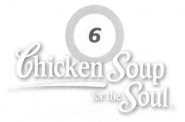

To Kingdom Come

Running made me feel like a bird let out of a cage, I loved it that much.
~Priscilla Welch

The Back Forty, I called it. I claimed it as mine.

Actually, the underdeveloped, underused property was part of the city's parklands and skirted the inside shoreline of the lake that belonged to the Greeley Irrigation Ditch Company. There wasn't even a discernible footpath when I first discovered it nearly three decades ago, but that didn't deter me. I made it my own.

Dodging tobacco-spitting grasshoppers, I pioneered the course and tugged a wagonload of toddlers towards the open arms of spreading cottonwoods and the Promised Land: a damp, deserted beach. Over time, the red Radio Flyer, with its jumble of spindly legs and flapping ponytails, flattened the thigh-high weeds and rutted a trail.

We romped along the lake, the kids and I, flapping our arms like the Canada geese that took umbrage and frantic flight at our intrusion. We waded the shallows; we wandered the shore; we built tea-party castles in the coarse sand. The only running I did was to chase and corral kids for the tiresome trek home.

But civilization encroached in the Back Forty at the same rate as the burgeoning population along Colorado's Front Range. Right before our eyes, a playground sprouted. A soccer field seeded. A sculpture park blossomed. And tendrils of a newly-poured concrete sidewalk wound through it all.

Although school now claimed all four of my children, I still heeded the siren call of the trail, more tempting than ever. I began walking two miles, every day, no matter what.

I walked whenever I could comfortably escape the demanding schedule of an active family. Sometimes, dewy dawn greeted me. On other days, falling dusk settled around my shoulders. The solitary ramblings nourished me and my pace quickened along with my enthusiasm.

I discovered a kingdom nestled against the parapets of the pristine Rockies, and I reigned as queen. I reveled in a bucolic realm of flowering crabapples, fragrant Russian olives, and lush lilacs. I nodded at the regal blue heron standing sentinel on a jutting boulder at the edge of the lake and giggled at court jesters—ebony coots sluicing the shoals, as endearing as wind-up toys. I measured the seasons and the years by comical goslings stumbling up rocky outcroppings, the annual roil of carp spawning in the spillway, and yawning ice holes drilled by hopeful fishermen.

Year after year, my speed-walking excursions kept me on track and in shape. Meanwhile, my kids raced out the door and on to college. Then, with an abruptness that shook me to my core, everything came to a halt.

My oldest child, a newly-minted college graduate, was critically injured by a drunk driver and on life support. Dazed, I sped to his side. I traded the wonders of the walking trail for the terrors of a trauma unit.

Distrustful of the rickety elevator system in Los Angeles' decrepit yet imposing County Hospital, I breached the battlements of dank stairwells to huff nine flights up—and counted each step that brought me closer to my comatose son. Day after day. Week after week. Then, one glorious day, I was sprinting up them to greet his re-entry to awareness.

A few months later, we returned home, my son and I, to face rehab and a hopeful future. Ready for some time alone, I slipped into my cross trainers and headed to the familiarity and comfort of the foot trail.

My own awareness sharpened in new appreciation. Had the lake always been so blue? The squirrels so frisky? The cottonwoods so towering? My steps quickened in eagerness—so quick, in fact, that I found myself jogging.

Loping.

Running.

Toned by the hospital stairwells and with a newfound leanness honed from stress, my body insisted on more than my old walking pace. More speed. A longer stride. A steady gait.

Flushed with exhilaration, I emptied my mind of the worries I'd accrued over the past several months. I freed myself from the dungeon of despair to focus on my breathing. I listened to my heartbeat. I felt my hamstrings stretch and the muscles in my calves elongate.

My arms pumped in automatic rhythm. A rhythm sure and even. A rhythm that consumed all thought and demanded a delightful focus. A rhythm that belonged only to me.

And so it began. An instant love of running.

Oh, a kernel of recognition rankled: I knew I wasn't cut from the same cloth as the marathoners who clogged the streets at the annual Lake-to-Lake event. I couldn't compete with the high school team that pounded the pavement to shape up for track meets. Even so, I ran. A middle-aged housewife, legs pumping, pulse pounding, sweat beading my brow—having the time of my life. I discovered a new, joyous pace. I reveled in the novelty. I understood the possibilities and delighted in the potential.

I ran.

I ran towards a hopeful future and the promising kingdom that beckoned.

~Carol McAdoo Rehme

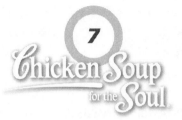

Dark Morning Running

I have to exercise in the morning before my brain figures out what I'm doing.
~Marsha Doble

In the Pacific Northwest during winter, 5:15 AM might as well be the dead of night. The alarm goes off and the only light is the red glow from my clock. My body says, "Go back to bed." But I don't. I know my running partner will be waiting in the street and I'm not going to stand her up. I drag myself into shoes and layers of moisture-wicking material plus hat, gloves, jacket and sometimes a scarf. Not only is it dark, it's cold.

I stumble onto the road, cursing the cold and wishing I were back under my warm covers. Yet I'm thankful most of the snow has melted, though some mornings, flurries still sting my face. Each carrying a flashlight, we meet between our houses. We chat as we run, setting off the motion-detecting porch lights as we go, and soon I'm warmer, awake and glad to be outside filling my lungs with quick breaths of cold air and putting one foot in front of the other, over and over again.

If you'd have asked me a year ago if I could see myself running at 5:15 on a winter morning I'd have laughed.

Morning just isn't my thing. Normally I need a double shot homemade latte and a bowl of cereal before I'm even functional and that's after 8:00 AM. So running in the morning was something I didn't even consider. "I prefer to work out midmorning or in the afternoon," I'd say to friends who go to the gym before work.

With a telecommuting job, I have the flexibility to work out at different times, but often I haven't. Many days I'd put on workout clothes first thing in the morning, with good intentions to run or do aerobics when I was more awake or had more energy or needed a break. But then those mornings would turn to evening with me still sitting at my computer working, without having worked out.

Then, last fall I reconnected with an old neighborhood friend. Our kids used to go to the same school and she only lives a couple of blocks away, but I hadn't seen her in over a year. She'd been running with a partner in the morning and taken off forty pounds that year. "Wow!" I said. When I looked in the mirror or got on the scale I knew I could benefit from the same kind of weight loss.

Since her running partner had gotten a treadmill and wasn't running outside, I found myself asking if I could join her. An inner voice screamed, "Are you crazy? You aren't a morning person." But I knew I needed to change something if I was ever going to get back in shape. I thought perhaps the accountability of a running partner might be it.

The first two months were especially hard, because we ran twice a week at 5:15 AM and I slept till 7:00 the other mornings. My body wasn't acclimating to the early hours and every run was difficult. Then it snowed and snowed and we took two months off. During the break I did a better job of working out at home, but I looked forward to the snow melting so we could resume our runs. I didn't miss the exercise so much as the chats and camaraderie. When the roads were clear enough we started up again, and soon were running together five days a week.

While some days it's still hard, most days it just feels normal. I even wake up a few minutes before the alarm now. And as I've adjusted to the routine of running I've discovered little joys that make it even more worthwhile than a little weight loss.

When the sky is clear I spot the Big Dipper and a host of sparkling stars. It reminds me of summertime camping and I look forward to running in warmer weather, without all these clothes.

We don't see many other runners in the wee hours, just one or two if any. On some routes we see more deer than people. Herds graze on the golf course and make nightly treks from the woods into the outlying neighborhoods. Sometimes they startle us when we glimpse their stationary shadowy figures. Sometimes we startle them and they go from a standing to a smooth sprint in seconds. We stop and watch for a moment, moving on when they are past. Oh, to run like a deer.

While we say "good morning" to those rare other runners, we can't even see their faces or make eye contact. And shining a flashlight in their eyes would be rude. But something about the craziness and camaraderie of running in the dark makes me feel like we are part of an exclusive club.

While I haven't lost forty pounds yet, it's amazing how much more energy I have, how much stronger I feel. It's the strange irony of rising early to run that the rest of the day is more productive than when I stayed in bed an extra hour or two. I wouldn't say I've become a morning person, but I would say morning running is now my thing.

~Jill Barville

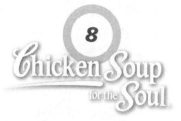

Taking a Leap of Faith

I can believe anything, provided that it is quite incredible.
~Oscar Wilde

Four short years ago, I rejoiced after escaping one of those dreaded 2-mile gym fitness runs. I hated running with a passion; it was just something that never came easily to me. As a short-statured, and somewhat stocky girl, I'd always been a back-of-the-pack runner who struggled to finish the very labored laps. At that time, if you had told me that I would one day run a marathon, I'd have told you in all honesty that I had a better chance of winning the lottery.

The turning point came when I met Mrs. Gray. I was in awe that she was fifty years old, going through chemotherapy for her recurring cancer, and still managed to run 30 miles a week. I figured that if Mrs. Gray could run 6 miles at a time, I could run at least one or two. In February, in the cold, bitter, Michigan weather, I started to walk a 2-mile route around my neighborhood and would struggle to add in short bursts of running. I'd start huffing and puffing, desperate to complete even a half-mile segment without stopping. Two months later, I finished the whole route, running, for the first time. I felt exhausted, but I felt incredible.

Over the next several years, I continued to push each run for a few extra minutes, slowly building my endurance. Those last few minutes would often be excruciating: my quads burning, my lungs begging for air, my mind wrestling against my body, ready to be done. Despite the physical and mental battle, I loved every minute of these runs—I knew I was not only building physical endurance, but also perseverance, mental strength, and a passion for running. A runner was born, and at 4'10" and 110 pounds, she was one who did not exactly fit the tall and thin ideal. It didn't matter to me; my heart was in it completely. I didn't need to compete against other runners, for my most important competition was myself.

After building a solid mileage base of about 25-30 miles per week, I started entering some local road races. Being an endurance runner, rather than one with speed, I was drawn toward the 10K races. Although I loved improving my times, nothing competed with the feeling of going into distances of "uncharted territory." After continuing to challenge myself and finishing two half marathons, I knew it was time to step it up. I decided I would train for the Detroit Free Press/Flagstar Bank Marathon.

My summer was filled with many long 6 AM runs in an effort to beat the brutal summer heat. Despite the labored last miles, painful quads, tight IT bands, necessary ice baths and compromised sleep, I loved my training. I knew I was finally on the road to conquering my "Everest." The prospect of crossing the finish line after running 26.2 miles helped me truly comprehend my capabilities.

Race day finally came, and I was filled with infinite excitement and apprehension. It was finally time to see what I was made of. With the gorgeous weather, scenic course, supportive Detroit and Windsor spectators, and the reality of my soon feat, the experience ended up being incredible. I did struggle through the last few miles, but after my journey, there was no doubt in my mind that I'd finish. As I crossed the finish line, I experienced the strongest sense of pride and happiness I ever had in my life. I was now a marathoner.

As John Bingham once said, "The miracle isn't that I finished. The miracle is that I had the courage to start."

~Marianne Mousigian

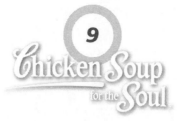

The Jogging Mommy

The coach's main job is 20 percent technical and 80 percent inspirational.
~Franz Stampfl

For the past thirty-odd years, my running career has consisted of mad dashes out the door, sprints to buses, and skillful hallway maneuvers to reach my desk on time. Sure, I did the required laps around the track in high school, but my heart was never in it. I kept a leisurely pace that allowed me to gossip with my classmates and protected my big 1980s hair from falling too much. Let's face it—asking much more from a teenage girl who is given only 5 minutes afterward to freshen up is just ridiculous.

Not that I'm anti-exercise. I have always enjoyed riding my stationary bike, doing aerobics, even bouncing around on a mini-trampoline in the living room. Jogging, however, was something in which I had no interest. As far as I was concerned, "runner's high" was some lofty promise started by marketers of athletic shoes.

My opinion of the activity began to change a bit when my husband decided to take it up last year. Heart disease runs in his family, and he wanted to really start pumping those coronary muscles. While I admired and encouraged his effort, I never expected it to last. Yet morning after morning, I would wake up to find him out pounding the pavement.

Our three-year-old son, Zachary, became intrigued by his father's morning ritual. Inevitably, he asked to tag along. His request was denied. Preschoolers cannot be trusted to run a straight path to any destination (except maybe when candy is involved), and exercise becomes too stressful when you are worrying about your child dashing into the street.

Zachary dropped the issue for many months, but it resurfaced the following summer. This time, it didn't seem like such a bad idea. Life in our area had been rather tough for the past few months. A rash of random shootings kept most of the neighborhood indoors in the fall (though my husband kept jogging, jokingly saying he was too fast to be caught), the winter was uncharacteristically harsh (and my husband jogged on the cleared streets), and spring showers made playgrounds a mess (and finally got my husband to use the exercise bike for a bit instead). A tad more outdoor activity would be good for the kid.

We decided on a track at a local school in order to avoid the traffic issue. I agreed to monitor Zachary so that my husband could exercise without interruption. Of course Zachary did not want to run alone, so I ended up jogging alongside.

Perhaps "jogging" is not the right word. First he did his best Carl Lewis imitation, followed by a dead stop to catch his breath. Then he wanted to walk and have me tell him stories. Then he suddenly left the tale about a giant to catch up to his dad. Then he strolled around with the water bottle. The stop-and-go lasted the entire time, and so did his smile.

At first I was rather annoyed by Zachary's lack of a plan. How were he and I supposed to count this as our daily exercise if it was so disorganized? I realized something though. Somewhere in there, we really did burn off some calories. Better yet, we also had fun.

Our sojourns continued for weeks. I felt my thighs and midsection getting firmer. I was out of breath less often, and at times I even left Zachary to wander the track by himself while I ran ahead (and kept a watchful eye). I was becoming (gulp) a runner.

On one particularly hot day, Zachary decided to get rid of his shirt. As sweat continued to pour down my neck, he asked me why I didn't do the same. Foolish child, I thought, you may have tricked me into running, but the last time I bared my midriff in the great outdoors was at a kiddy pool at age two. My husband sided with him.

I figured, what the heck, I'll humor them once (I had a sports top on underneath my T-shirt).

The result was unexpected. I didn't feel stupid—I felt free. The wind felt wonderful against my newly exposed skin, and I felt like an athlete instead of a mother trying to cover up her body. My husband's approval and a glance or two from some other males did not hurt either. And who had time to worry about showing the world that I was not a supermodel when there was running to do?

The real test of my commitment to jogging came later in the summer when Zachary started morning day camp. There was no way we could be done jogging and showering by the time it started each day. Our family ritual had to end, but my own began.

Clad in my serious-looking sportswear, I kept going to the track. I figured my workout would be different without a toddler along, but it really was much the same (minus the stories about giants). I walked. I ran. I didn't count laps. When I was tired, I quit. I, too, left the track smiling. I guess the old saying of kids changing you in ways you never thought possible is true. I never would have imagined my son being the best coach I ever had.

~Beth Braccio Hering

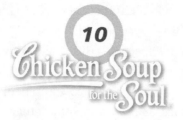

Who Knew?

I decided to go for a little run.
~Forrest Gump

I've always been more academic than athletic. Throughout middle school and high school, I was heavily involved in student council and the Honor Society. And no sports whatsoever.

But at least one physical education course was required for high school graduation. And being able to run a mile—without dying—was required to pass said P.E. course. I know I sound like a complete wimp, but I rarely, if ever, ran by choice, let alone raced around the quarter-mile track four times.

To be honest, I didn't think I could do it. But if I wanted to graduate, I had to try.

The P.E. teacher explained that we would have two weeks to train before our big run. The first day I barely made it around the track once before I was breathing into a paper sack. Pathetic. But after a week of training, I was able to jog two laps before I needed my lunch bag respirator. And on the last day of our training period, I was able to complete the required four laps. It certainly wasn't pretty, but I did it. I was the slowest one in the whole class, but lucky for me, the only time limit was the fifty-minute class period.

I just had to do it again the next day to earn my P.E. credit. No problem, I thought. If I can do it once, I can do it a second time. What I didn't count on was the audience.

The co-ed audience.

Oh, the humiliation, I thought as I squatted down at the starting line. Patrick, the boy I'd liked for the past three years, was sitting in the bleachers. The boys' gym classes were going to use the track after our big race.

Just completing the mile was no longer enough. Now, with Patrick watching, I had to look good doing it.

The first lap wasn't too bad. I kept up with the pack—sort of. During the second lap, I fell behind—way behind. But on the third lap, I was back with the pack—yes, they'd lapped me. My fourth lap was utterly humiliating. I was the only one on the track, huffing and puffing and praying that I would cross the finish line before I hyperventilated. In the home stretch, I looked up into the bleachers and noticed that the boys were no longer sitting there. Patrick was not witnessing my fourth lap horror. Oh, joy!

The next day in chemistry class, Patrick grinned at me and said, "You looked good running yesterday. Why don't you go out for the cross country team?"

I looked at him like he was from Mars. "Running isn't my thing," I said.

"Really? When I saw you yesterday in gym class, you were running next to Jenny and Tina, and they're the team's fastest girls."

Now I knew he was from Mars.

"So, in what place did you end up?" he continued. "I had homework to do and I only saw a few minutes of the race."

"You didn't see the end?"

Patrick shook his head. "So what happened? You started off so strong."

I gulped, unsure of what to say. As I debated how to answer, he said, "You know, I'd really like to see you try out for the team. It's a total blast." He put his hand on mine and added, "I'll even give you a ride home after practice. Maybe we can stop for a burger on the way."

I felt my face flush. Had Patrick just asked me out? My dreams were coming true. And all I had to do was join the cross country team.

So, for love, I did. But there was just one problem. Eventually,

Patrick was going to watch me run for more than 10 seconds and when he did, he'd realize the truth about my athletic abilities. I sucked.

I wanted to impress Patrick and make him like me. And this seemed to be strongly linked to me not sucking at running long distances. So I started practicing. I ran before school, and after school, and on the weekends. Sometimes I ran until I felt like my lungs would explode. But they never did—and somehow, I began to enjoy that feeling. I actually started looking forward to my runs.

And just a few weeks later, the ride home in Patrick's car was no longer the best thing about cross country practice. Patrick was nice, and I liked him. But the truth was that I'd come to love running.

Patrick and I fizzled out when the cross country season ended, but my infatuation with running has become a life-long affair.

Who knew?

~Diane Stark

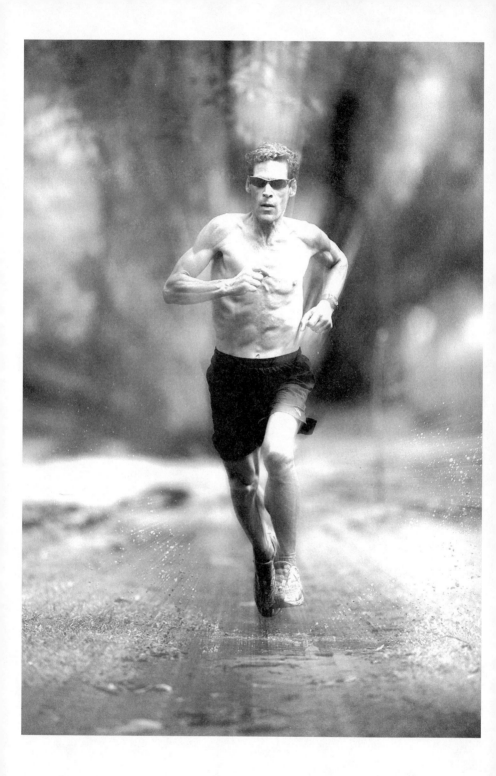

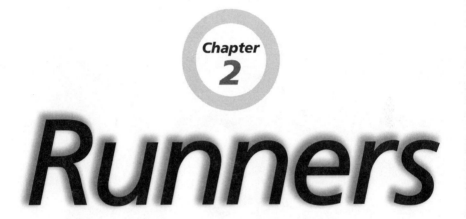

Chapter 2

Runners

Running Therapy

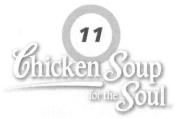

The Sanctity of the Run

Sweat cleanses from the inside.
It comes from places a shower will never reach.
~George Sheehan

I ran competitively as a teenager. I was the daughter of a struggling single parent, and running was my escape from a broken home and the burden of never having enough money. Running was relatively cheap, and it took me places I would not have gone otherwise. I was even banking on a track scholarship to get me through college since my mom, then working as a minimum-wage clerk, clearly couldn't afford my tuition.

Then, at the beginning of my senior year, I was in a terrible car accident. Before I knew it, I was stranded in a hospital bed with a shattered lumbar, a cracked pelvis, a punctured lung, and several broken ribs. Needless to say, the accident quelled my dreams.

But life moved on, as it always does. My body slowly healed, and I struggled to finish high school and carve out a new identity for myself and forge new hobbies. I eventually worked my way through college, got married, and began having a family, another deep aspiration of mine. Growing up for the most part alone, I yearned for a home full of the bustle of family life.

As a mother of five, my life has moved from the open trail into the kitchen in a race to get meals whipped up before children begin a hunger howl. When I want to go running, I have to sneak out of my house. It's a rapid-fire affair of throwing on workout clothes (clean or otherwise), lacing up shoes as I'm going out the door, and darting off without anyone (except Dad) noticing I'm gone. The youngest of my brood gets miffed if he notices Mommy leaving without his approval or companionship.

I don't marathon run. I don't have a schedule or a ritual. For me, I usually look around the house and think, "Okay, everything's under control here… It's nice outside… I'm going running." And I dash off. I'm not training for official races; I'm training for my life.

I try to run three or four times a week. Aside from the obvious health reasons, I run to keep sane. I knew I wanted to be a mother, but I didn't know love in a big package comes with a price tag: emotional and mental instability. There's something grounding about the steady rhythm of my feet hitting the pavement accompanied by the sound of my breathing that is close to music—close to meditation.

My house is a bustling den of undone chores. There's always that load of laundry that begs to be done and a meatloaf that needs to be made. There's always a diaper to change, a floor to mop, an argument to mediate, and a missing toy to find. And, if I still have time, there's a bathroom that needs my attention.

The demands can be overwhelming at times. I love my family immensely, but I don't love getting hit in the head with a phone by a baby who's just learned to use his arm. I love my boys, but I tire of piles of smelly socks and scattered unmentionables. I don't mind cleaning my house, but I do grow weary of toothpaste smeared lavishly on bathroom mirrors and unidentifiable sticky spots showing up on freshly-mopped kitchen floors.

So, when I'm feeling especially anxious and irritated, I take off. I run. Sometimes I run hard and fast, pumping my arms to push up hills as if to punish myself (or to escape a dog). Sometimes I jog slowly and luxuriously, enjoying the scent of blossoming peach trees and the feel of a spring breeze, or taking in the heavy wet scent of an approaching storm.

Sometimes when I run, I look up, enjoying puffy clouds, a glaring sun, or the ominous darkness of approaching storm clouds. Sometimes I look out at the horizon—at the mountains blanketed in a green that never goes away—and I am happily reminded of my diminutive existence. Sometimes I look down because of dangers lurking in the form of potholes, loose gravel, or stray rocks. Sometimes I delightedly notice lizards crossing my path or butterflies resting silently on oleander bushes. I see children riding their bikes, elderly couples walking their dogs, women in pairs wearing colorful track suits, walking and chatting. With all of these observations, I am reminded of the wonders of the world and the steady existence of life beyond whatever small calamity befalls mine.

When I get myself into a rhythm of striding and breathing, I begin to feel the invisible, heavy layers of stress shed. I leave them behind to eat my dust, and I am a lighter being, pushing on ahead. By the end of my run, I am wet with perspiration, my heart is beating rapidly, and I am feeling new and alive.

My life as a mother is like an endurance sport. My runs always remind me of what life is: always putting one foot in front of the other, even when I'm exhausted. It's about running up the hill, however daunting, and congratulating myself for not stopping. Life, like running, is about getting up and pushing on ahead, even if I've tripped on a pothole. It's about keeping the rhythm and setting a pace. It's about minding my injuries and allowing myself time to heal, but not letting injuries get the best of me. Running is like life; it is a glorious, albeit sometimes painful, act of always moving forward.

When I finish my runs, I return home happily to the energy and bustle of my lovely family. My house seems warmer and friendlier. My children are chatting and playing, and I smile and hold them close. They tell me they missed me and wonder where I ran. I tell them I've missed them, as well.

I feel refreshed, grounded, and sane. I feel victorious. My mind is clear and my heart is happy. Everything is right with the world, and I'm ready to tackle that laundry pile and scrub that bathroom.

~Luci L. Creery

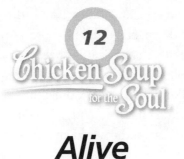

Alive

Running is real. It's all joy and woe, hard as diamond.
It makes you weary beyond comprehension, but it also makes you free.
~Jesse Owens

I was born with very poor eyesight. Retinitis pigmentosa limited what I could do to a certain degree. Night blindness prevented me from doing a lot of things after dark. Sometimes I felt like a restless tiger trapped in a cage. There was a whole jungle out there to explore, and I couldn't get to all of it.

I had to sit close to the TV to see what was going on. At school it was hard seeing the chalkboard and I usually sat in the front row. If I sat in the back with my friends, they would tell me what to write. Steps and bleachers were difficult, almost terrifying, for me, and I navigated them cautiously. I thought there was something wrong with me because I couldn't bound up and down them the way my friends and classmates did.

Now I know why. My depth perception and peripheral vision were terrible.

Close activities, like reading, writing, and sketching, were things at which I excelled.

And running.

As much as I liked indoor activities, I was an outdoor tomboy too. Climbing trees, riding bikes, playing with my dog.

And running.

Running was something that didn't require fine visual acuity. If I knew where the finish line was, I was there.

Speed is a gift. I didn't know why I was blessed with speed when I was a young girl, but I was. My dad said I could run like a deer, and I did. But not in track. Our small rural school didn't have track. It was in P.E. I was faster than all the girls, and faster than all the boys except for one, who was a basketball player.

Maybe this was God's way of making it up to me?

I liked it.

It felt good to run. To be faster than everyone. To win.

It felt like flying. It felt free.

I didn't need good vision to run fast.

Even then, I recognized it as something special. Power surged in my legs, muscles, lungs, bones, brain, soul. It was a natural high.

Running kept my self-esteem going. With it came a keen sense of the physicality of my own body. I had trouble with the stairs, but on the gym floor or in the field, or in a yard, it was a different story.

Pride — the good kind of pride — swelled inside me each time I came in first.

It was effortless.

Some of my classmates could sing, play the piano, sew clothes.

I ran.

When running laps around the gym floor, I would often pass my classmates a couple of times.

The farm I grew up on provided wide open spaces to explore and have fun. Lots of room for running.

My vision continued to deteriorate over the years, but my runner's high didn't. The strength and self-esteem it generated carried me through some challenging times — single parenthood, college, grad school, the loss of a man, the loss of one career due to my eyesight, the start of another....

I was never, never a professional runner. Never in organized sports. The trophy on my dresser is the one my son Travia got in T-ball. The medals awarded to me are two college degrees.

In a way I'm glad running didn't become a sport for me, or part of an exercise regimen, or something I did for a living. It served a much different and personal purpose. The spirituality of it influenced me far more than my other talents and skills. It allowed me to experience success early. It showed me who I was and what I could do. It let me feel victory.

Were it not for running, I might not have met life's challenges or pursued my dreams.

This may be another reason for my blessing of speed and strength: For what lay ahead. All my resources were called on to navigate life's stair steps.

For me, the runner's high has lasted a lifetime. It reached far beyond the moment when my legs were pumping and my muscles were thrumming and my brain was soaring.

It even reaches into my sleep at night, because sometimes I still have dreams where I'm running fast and free. My heart pounds, my breath quickens, my muscles thrive.

I guess not everyone understands this. But a runner will.

~Tammy Ruggles

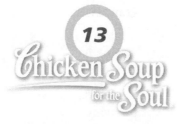

The Secret

O public road, I say back I am not afraid to leave you, yet I love you,
you express me better than I can express myself.
~Walt Whitman

I'm not as confident as I seem
But the road doesn't know that
It simply is
Hard and smooth beneath my shoes
As I start my morning run

I'm not as sure as I seem
But the road doesn't know that
It stretches out before me
Like a string of unbroken promises
A morning just ready to begin

I'm not as strong as I seem
But the road doesn't know that
It waits for me like a familiar friend
Nonjudgmental, yet
All-knowing

I hurt, I ache, I mourn
But the road doesn't know that
Nor does it care
It simply is

Every day the same, a constant star
This I know for sure

I can't go any farther
But the road doesn't know that
It beckons me on, encouraging me
To break my record
Test my limits
Prove to myself I can do better

That's the secret
between the road and I

~Tina Bausinger

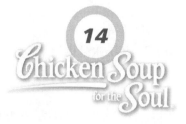

Moving Forward

We will continue to invent the future through our blood and tears and through all our sadness.... We will prevail....
~Nikki Giovanni,
Virginia Tech University Distinguished Professor, poet

I've gone running here hundreds of times. My feet were on the same pavement, passing the same buildings, navigating the same course. This time, though, something was starkly different.

It wasn't the air hanging heavy in my lungs and it wasn't the unseasonably cold weather—flurries in mid-April. It was my heart.

Physically, everything was normal. For once, moving blood and oxygen through my body was the least of my heart's worries. As a runner I can ignore soreness, snow storms, injuries and cramps, but the pain of running at Virginia Tech after the tragic shootings in April 2007 was something I could not simply grit my teeth and run through.

Virginia Tech is a safe place; no one can convince me otherwise. Not my countless friends who lectured me on the dangers of running alone at night on a college campus, and not Cho Seung-Hui, who killed thirty-two students and teachers before turning the gun on himself.

I graduated from Virginia Tech almost exactly three years before the school became nationally-known for the shooting. After graduation I packed up my apartment and put on my running shoes for one last run in Blacksburg.

Virginia Tech is on a 26,000-acre campus surrounded by

breathtaking trails and rolling pastures. Despite the call of the trail, my favorite run was always right on campus, usually at night. Long after the sun set behind the Blue Ridge Mountains I darted between buildings, dodged students and reveled in the moonlit academic landscape.

Somewhere between football games, homework and sleep deprivation, running almost immediately found its place in my life at Virginia Tech. I still remember my first run as a freshman. Just hours after my mom and dad moved me into my freshman dorm, West Ambler-Johnston (the dorm where Emily Hilscher and Ryan Hall were killed), a few friends from high school and I jogged around campus, exploring our new home. A few nights later I embarked on the campus on my own and discovered a beautiful sanctuary that I somehow missed while walking to classes.

In college I grew from a mediocre high school miler who was secretly intimidated by the distance of a 5K into a confident half-marathoner and triathlete. The hours I spent on campus in my running shoes were the only time I knew for sure what I wanted to do with my life: I wanted to be a runner.

Sitting in my office at a newspaper three hours from Blacksburg, the initial news of the shootings hit me like a blow to the knees. I frantically called my brother, a freshman at Tech, and choked on tears as I watched the death toll climb. Just hours later my editor sent me to Blacksburg to cover the story.

Being back on campus amidst the mourning, the media and the yellow tape caused stress deeper than any exam ever had. I spent the afternoon focusing on work rather than the reality of what was happening around me. I conducted interviews, took photos and went to press conferences.

Eventually, though, the sun set on that April day, and when my first round of stories were sent the reality of the tragedy at my beloved college began to sink in. Before a lump could form in my throat I pulled my hair into a ponytail, slipped on my running shoes and started running.

That night, forward motion was laborious. In the stillness of campus, where I remembered feeling fast and strong, my legs felt heavy and my muscles burdened. Instead of listening to my reluctant body I fixed my gaze ahead, determined to take each step. As the Drillfield, a large grassy field in the center of campus, came into view, my feet instinctively stopped. The field where students play Frisbee and pick-up football had been transformed into a vigil and was glowing with the mournful warmth of candles. Suddenly, I couldn't ignore it anymore. The rush of emotion overwhelmed me and I bent over with my hands on my knees. Then, just like that, as my breaths were overtaken by sobs, I started running again. Tears streamed down my face as I circled the Drillfield. I was angry to the core and overwhelmed with sadness. I cried for the victims, for the survivors, for the campus, for myself, and I ran because I didn't know what else to do. Soon my weary muscles felt powerful, my breaths were strong and my steps were sure. As I ran, the strength of my alma mater fueled each step.

I rounded the Drillfield and paused at Norris Hall, where most of the shootings took place. The building was encircled by police tape and patrol cars. My feet slowed, but they did not stop. I didn't stop because I couldn't. Virginia Tech taught me about progress and the importance of moving forward. For years the energy I felt on the campus of Virginia Tech and the spirit of the Hokies fueled my runs. Virginia Tech never let me stop and now, more than ever, stopping was not an option.

Running at Virginia Tech got me through exams, heartbreak, and all of the trials that come with becoming an adult. My runs taught me what the classroom couldn't: that no pain lasts as long as you think it will, that I can go about twice as far as I first thought I could and it taught me that even when everything is going wrong, it is possible to be strong.

~Amanda Southall

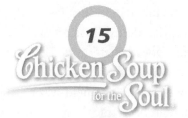
Changing Course

Running gives freedom. When you run you can determine your own tempo.
You can choose your own course and think whatever you want.
~Nina Kuscik: marathon runner

I quit running on November 26, 2005. My last run had been a rolling five-mile loop along backcountry roads in the drizzling rain. Occasionally a house broke the tree line or a car sped past, but the world was silent, calm, mine. My legs were light; I had shed my life's stresses and worries at the door like an extra layer of fleece on a warm day. They were, however, waiting for me when I returned.

I opened the front door 50 minutes later. My brother, Kevin, greeted me. He sat in the green, overstuffed recliner in the corner, the same chair he had slept in for the past several weeks. "Did you have fun?" he asked. He couldn't lift his head off his chest, only raised his eyebrows and glanced in my direction. Kevin was dying of cancer. Lung cancer, actually, but tumors had taken his eyesight, moved to his brain, and had begun burrowing into his spinal cord. The scar from last spring's brain surgery stretched across the top of his shaved head and frowned at me. Scabs from the summer's radiation oozed and puddled on his scalp. The doctor had sentenced him to fourteen months of life; he was in his sixth.

The smile smeared across my face vanished. Guilt pinned me to the floor. The exhilaration, the high from the perfect run, drained from my body and seemed to pool at my feet, mixing with the rainwater that dripped from my shirt and hair. I managed to mumble, "Yeah, it was good."

I quit running that day. It wasn't fair for me to lace up my Brooks when my thirty-six-year-old brother could barely cross a room without wheezing. So, for seven months, through chemotherapy, radiation, and doctor visits, I visualized running up and down the hills along Route 522 on our way to Geisinger Hospital in Danville, Pennsylvania. I lay in bed at night listening to Kevin's raspy breathing while I thought of the various marathons and road races I'd finished over the years. Thoughts of running nagged me, but I refused to give in and take those precious steps out the door that led to a run, an escape.

Kevin, however, was running a marathon that promised no medal at the finish, only rest and relief. He passed away on July 7, 2006. There were no grand revelations, no life altering ah-ha's, just loss. His life ended and mine trudged on. I needed comfort; I needed to run, to leave behind the grief and hopelessness wrought by the cancer.

My first run came a week after his passing. I ran the same loop that I had ended with seven months earlier. This time I ran it backwards as if I were searching for a pair of lost keys. I was searching for the passion I had left on the slopes and sharp bends. My legs were heavy and slow, but the pain let me know I was alive. It was hot and I cried through the first mile and a half.

I run slower now, and most runs start with thoughts of my brother, but now I run because he can't. Running never leaves us. It just changes course sometimes.

~Jennifer Freed

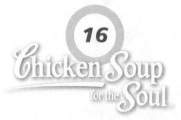

Running Meditation

Move and the way will open.
~Zen Proverb

I t was a couple of weeks after midterm during the second semester of my first college year when the stress really started to hit me. The difficulty of my classes was not in itself enough to faze me, but combined with increased responsibilities at work, financial worries, and my own perfectionism that would settle for nothing less than an A in any subject, my nerves were completely shot. I had tried meditation many times, but with minimal success. It is not in my nature to sit for long and I was having a rough time focusing on my breath with my mind so full of x+y and the endless stream of exams. It became an effort just to get out of bed in the morning. That is until one day a friend from class suggested that I take up running.

She had been diagnosed the year before with diabetes, and as a result, her doctor recommended that she lose some weight. She had initially taken up running with that goal in mind. She was startled after only a couple of months to find that the benefits of the exercise far exceeded shedding a few pounds. She insisted that after a run she felt more alert, more energetic and less stressed out in general. "Just try it. Twenty minutes a day and I guarantee it will change your life."

"Twenty minutes," I replied, "I'm lucky if I have 5 minutes to brush my teeth. I just don't have the time."

"Make the time," she said. So I did.

The idea of running did appeal to me. I like to be active and I had always wanted to give it a try. Since nerves usually woke me before my alarm in the mornings anyway I figured that instead of lying awake for half an hour fretting over quizzes, I could at least make constructive use of the time.

Following her advice I started out slowly, 20 minutes alternating jogging and walking, then gradually working my way up a full twenty-minute run. I started out around 5 AM, and I think it was the peace of those waking hours that initially kept me in the routine. I loved the stillness of the town at that hour, when the only sounds were the birdsongs and my own footsteps treading along the path. I had never watched a sunrise until then and I was mesmerized by the steady transformation of night into day.

In the beginning, it was all I could to do to keep my breath flowing. I learned quickly that I had to develop a rhythm in my breathing if I was going to achieve any reasonable distance. I also had to make this rhythm coincide with my body's movements. It was mind and body working together, a complete harmony achieved through consistency and focus. I was exhilarated by this newfound sense of balance. For what felt like the first time in my life I felt clear about something. I felt stable and at the same time I felt free.

During my jog I would first focus on my stride and then, once I felt steady, I would just focus on my breath, simply letting it flow in and out in its own natural rhythm. I let my thoughts come and go, holding onto nothing, just watching my breath. It took me a while to realize that what I was doing was actually a form of meditation. By that time I had already begun to notice its effects in my daily life.

I found myself not dwelling so much on work and school and increasing piles of bills, but on matters far outside the daily trials of life, like the natural rhythms that take place all around us. The natural flow of life that we often fail to notice in our eternal rush. During my run I would observe the seasonal changes and the way the plants and animals would adjust accordingly and I would feel connected to it all.

I also noticed that I didn't feel so tense anymore. I still had my moments of worry, but I stopped feeling consumed by them. I felt stronger, physically and mentally. I laughed more and studied less for the simple fact that I felt more able to retain the information quickly and in greater detail than ever before. As I began to challenge myself while running I also learned to meet complications in my life in a similar manner. I would try my best and if I made it, great, if not I would keep at it until I did. I came to understand that one setback does not equal failure.

I usually run up to an hour each day now. I can't imagine my life without it. I love the feeling it gives me, a feeling I am still learning to carry with me throughout the day. It is my meditation, my gateway to that space inside that we all need to go to at some point in the day. That space where we are able to tune out the world, if only for a moment, and allow ourselves to just be.

~Cristina M. Cherry

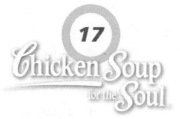

The Marathon Miracle

Miracles happen to those who believe in them.
~Bernard Berenson

It's 6:15 in the morning and the pavement is flying beneath me. With each stride through the dark, frosty morning, I'm gobbling up yards of San Vicente Boulevard as I head for the final stretch back to the office. Even though I'm cold and clammy, there's a certain exhilaration knowing that there aren't many others up at this hour, let alone preparing for an event like the marathon: 26.2 miles of grueling, energy-sapping punishment.

I had wanted to run a marathon for more than twenty years. But even during the fog of my alcohol and drug addiction, I somehow acknowledged that subjecting my body to the rigors of long-distance running would be a more expedient death than a bottle or another line of coke. But, when I finally got clean and sober on October 21, 1986, the world opened up to me. For the first time in my life, goals and aspirations seemed within reach without the artificial obstacles of youth, immaturity or my own physical and mental limitations. I could do anything I put my mind to.

Ironically, what complicated the issue was my college degree — in particular, my area of study. In 1983, I graduated from San Diego State University with a degree in Exercise Physiology and went to work for a cardiac rehabilitation clinic. My denial allowed me to drink to excess every night while I counseled patients on the value of taking care of one's health by day. For the next several years, every patient that I came in contact with naturally assumed that I was the picture of health and a marathoner. After all, haven't all exercise physiologists completed at least one? I struggled with my disease while in my own mind I felt invalidated as a fitness expert who was touting the benefits of a healthy lifestyle.

When I finally entered recovery, I had no excuses or limitations. I was determined to go for it. Over the next six months, I read every conceivable book on the subject of marathon training. I experimented with everything from diet, running shoes, shorts and fluid replacements—even underwear. Every Saturday morning was reserved for my long runs (between 15 and 25 miles) while the weekdays were peppered with shorter hill climbs and weight training. As the mileage and dirty laundry piled up, I became a fit and highly-tuned running machine.

With one week to go before the Los Angeles Marathon, short cruising runs were the order of the day; the concept being after months of preparation, it's time to cruise and relax. Just keep limber and get ready for the big race on Sunday.

As I approached the final stretch of my pre-dawn run, out of nowhere a pothole suddenly appeared, dropping me to the asphalt. On the way down, I heard an audible "pop" from my left knee. In one split second, six months of training evaporated in the wake of my dislocated knee. By the time I hobbled back to the office, it had swollen to the size of a cantaloupe.

While I wasn't immediately sure just how badly I was injured, I had taken enough anatomy classes to know that knees were not supposed make sounds and look like cantaloupes. But the thought of missing the marathon in five days concerned me far more than my physical infirmity. I had not just given the marathon a small place in my life; it had become my life. I had shared all of my competitive dreams of running my first marathon in my hometown with my friends and everyone else who was important in my life. Now my dream was gone.

I managed to see an orthopedic surgeon the next day, having already lost one valuable day of training. For the uninitiated, losing a single day of training when preparing for a marathon begins a downward spiral that can potentially erode the confidence necessary to complete a race that defies the limits of common sense. Lying on the exam table with a synovial fluid-filled syringe protruding from the side of my knee was not exactly instilling the type of pre-race confidence that I had hoped for.

The good news was that after a thorough examination, X-rays and an MRI, nothing appeared to be permanently damaged. When I stepped into the pre-dawn rut, I stretched every ligament, tendon and joint capsule to the extent of their unnatural limits; but nothing was broken. The first thing I asked the doctor was, "When will I be able to run again?" Remaining cautious, he explained that as soon as the swelling went down, I could do whatever I felt I could tolerate. The gauntlet was thrown down.

Later that afternoon, my self-confidence began to return to normal, even though my knee hadn't. The injury damaged my body, but not my spirit. The next day, I hobbled into a local running store and asked if there were any marathons later in the year. With all of the training that I had put in, I was certain that I'd be back on the streets within a couple of months.

"There aren't any more marathons until the last part of November," said the clerk. "Oh, wait. There is one smaller race next month: the Long Beach Marathon." A ray of hope emerged.

Even despite the rosy picture the orthopedic surgeon painted, I was convinced as I limped along on my gammy leg that there was no way I could pursue the Long Beach Marathon. It was only three and a half weeks away. Impossible. But, Aristotle once said, "Hope is a waking dream." My dream was only three weeks away.

Fortunately, due to my area of study, I knew more about physiology than the average weekend athlete. I knew that if I could sustain my fitness at its current level while my knee mended, there was a possibility that I could run the race and maybe even finish it.

The next morning, I embarked on a self-prescribed training regimen unlike any you'll read about in *Runner's World*; probably the first time anyone has ever prepared for a marathon without running. I was fortunate enough to be working in a hospital fitness center that had a wide variety of stationary bikes, treadmills and free weights. One of the bikes was a Schwinn Airdyne, arguably one of the finest pieces of fitness equipment ever invented. The Airdyne is an over-sized contraption that has not only pedals, but arm cranks that thrust up from the flywheel. With a large fan mounted in front of the rider, the faster that you pedal the greater the resistance. Hmmm... This could actually work.

I hooked myself up with a series of electrocardiograph leads designed to monitor the heart rate and rhythm of cardiac patients during exercise. Having already calculated my training heart rate range based on my previous program, I knew that I could theoretically maintain my fitness if I could persevere through 90 minutes a day at a minimum of 150-165 beats per minute. I dragged a barstool up next to the bike and propped my ice-packed knee on it and proceeded to pedal with my good leg and both arms until I reached 150 beats per minute.

Over the course of the next week, I downed prescription-strength anti-inflammatories like candy. The swelling in my knee went down as my fitness level climbed. I was actually becoming fitter without putting in so much as a mile of running. After about two and a half weeks, I solicited the doctor's approval to start running again. He gave it.

The first day back out on the street was torture. I was handicapped more by my mental fitness than physical. After a few easy miles, I returned to the office with renewed confidence that I just might be able to finish my first marathon.

Within a week, I was back up to 10 miles. The Long Beach Marathon was now only days away. At a time when I should have been tapering down, I was ramping up. Trainers advise anyone contemplating running a marathon to run at least one run of 20 miles or more before the event. Fortunately, I had already completed mine, so I just considered my injury a minor "interruption" in my training schedule.

By the time race day arrived, I was fit and motivated to run the race of a lifetime. I completed the race in just under four hours, running the first 18 miles faster than I had ever run before. As I crossed the finish line, the loudspeakers announced my name and hometown to the crowd of cheering spectators. I immediately broke down in tears as the preceding seven months of stress finally oozed out of every pore of my body. I could finally relax; I had completed the Long Beach Marathon.

Over the next few years, I completed three more marathons, but none of those victories was a sweet as the first. The power to overcome overwhelming odds to attain an impossible goal made it even better than if my training had gone exactly as planned.

~Allen R. Smith

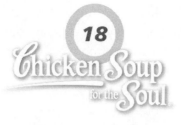

Full Circle

The wheel is come full circle, I am here.
~William Shakespeare

"I'm going for a run," I said loudly as I went out the door and down the stairs of the apartment where my mother, brothers and I lived. I was in a bad mood, and needed to get out of the house, to put as much distance as I could between my family and me. Things were pretty bad as far as my relationship with my mom and brothers was concerned. As a teenager I kept to myself and seemed to find fault with everything they said or did. We were all trying to make things work, but the pressure of trying to support each other through some very hard times was beginning to get to me.

So I began running. At first I would just take long walks to get away from everyone and everything. But the pressures and worries that filled my head and heart seemed to stay with me on those walks. I couldn't seem to shake the feeling that my family was falling apart and that I was only making things worse. My classes were a burden that I could hardly bear, and the part-time job I held at a donut shop felt like a dead end to me.

One day I just couldn't take it. I ran. I ran down the street and across the block and past another block and another. When I couldn't run anymore I stopped to catch my breath, bending over and feeling my chest heave with the effort of my crazy dash. Then I noticed that my head was clear, and that I hadn't thought about anything negative while I was running. So the next time I stormed out of the house and went for a walk I ran halfway through it. I ran until all thoughts of home and family and the miserable situation we were in faded from my consciousness. I found my mind clear and settled. I had found an answer. So I started running.

Things at home and at school and work didn't seem to get any better. As a matter of fact things seemed to get worse, as I pulled almost totally away from the people around me. My running became my release from all the stress and negative feelings I connected with my family. I went out running almost every day, no matter what the weather was like. If a day at home was really bad I'd go out more than once. There were days that I had to run and run and run to leave my problems behind. It was an escape that I turned to again and again.

Then one night I reached the lowest point in my life. I argued with my mom and brothers over things I should have been trying to help make better. Instead I blamed them for everything, and swore I was never coming back again. I went out and ran longer and faster than I'd ever run before. I ran until my lungs were on fire and I could barely see past the sweat that poured down my face. Overhead the moon followed me like a giant, unblinking eye.

Clouds rolled by. It started to rain. I ran past houses where soft lights shone through curtains and I could see people moving about. I imagined the families inside those houses laughing and listening to each other, offering help and hope to one another. I ran past the little neighborhood church where my mom liked to go on Sundays, and remembered how her last prayer at the end of each service was for her family. I ran past a couple walking the other way, holding hands and whispering to each other. The look on their faces was one of love and devotion. I ran on and on.

But this time instead of running until I could run no more and then stopping and slowly making my way back, I found that I'd run in a huge circle around the neighborhood, covering the endless blocks, the rain-slicked streets right back to my apartment. As I stood breathing heavily I looked through the living room window of the apartment, watching the shadows of my family as they moved about, picking up the pieces I'd left behind. I stood and thought about all the good memories, all the joy that existed there because of the love we had for each other. I realized I had to stop running from my problems, that I was responsible for helping my family, and that I needed to give them the love and support that I was looking for in them. I went back upstairs, listening to the sounds of the voices on the other side of the door, knowing I could make each voice a little happier, take away some of the sadness, if I tried hard enough.

Things got better. Those times that often seemed like they would never end changed, and our family grew closer as we held each other together. I still run. But now I run to think about all the wonderful people and the gifts that fill my life. I run to come back full circle to those challenges, those frustrations, those blessings and miracles that are mine to make the best of, not run away from. I run because I have a destination now: Home, and everyone there who's waiting for me.

~John P. Buentello

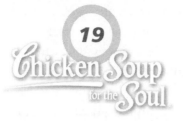

19

To Celebrate

There is no satisfaction without a struggle first.
~Marty Liquori

"We need to talk," my husband Michael stated as he woke me up.

Even though I was in a hazy state, the tone of his voice and words indicated something serious. Normally, he would sneak into our bed after his restaurant shift, letting his presence be known by the combined smells of cigarettes and alcohol. That night he didn't and it terrified me.

Our marriage was not the best during that time. We were like two ships passing. Our work schedules conflicted—my shift days and his nights. The phone became our sole connection as we called to check in with each other. He was working as the assistant manager of a restaurant, making a great salary with some perks, namely alcohol. The restaurant closed but the staff would stay and drink—and head out to other bars. To him, home meant sleeping it off and arguing with me about his habits. No, it was not the marriage we envisioned, but it was what we had—a faint connection to each other.

So there we sat on a tiny concrete balcony. He lit a cigarette and began to speak. He was being transferred. The promised general manager's position he coveted was given to the boss's relative. He knew his drinking was heavy and he was tired of fighting.

"It may be time to quit my job. What should I do?" he asked.

An immediate sense of relief washed over me; we were okay. I gave him the only answer I had. "What ever you feel is right." He tendered his resignation the next day. He cleared the house of alcohol that night. He quit smoking the next week.

Things got worse before they got better. He worked a handful of jobs, each a disappointment. It was hard on him, every interview leading to quizzical looks when they noted his management experience. They could not comprehend why someone would leave a high-paying career to work elsewhere. Eventually, he was hired at a lawn company. He left early each morning to pick up his list of houses. He was too good at it. The harder he worked the more houses they assigned. To make matters worse, the company equipment and truck were always malfunctioning. Every shift became a battle. Whenever I suggested that he quit, his pride prevailed: "I will do whatever it takes to support this family."

I finally received the dreaded call. He had broken down emotionally and couldn't do it anymore. He was found at the side of the road crying and heaving. The lawn company was called to pick up their vehicle; he would not be driving it again. The next week was spent in a haze of antidepressants and worry. I vividly remember taking a long walk together and doing most of the talking. He held my hand but remained silent and stared off into the distance. I was terrified that he was lost, racked with guilt that I had not seen this coming. Was it us? Was it me? "You are the only thing keeping me going," he reassured me.

Truthfully, I do not know how it happened; I just remember standing at the store financing the treadmill. He decided to run. He was taken aback at first; it was harder than he thought. Every day he would struggle against those taunting red lights on the machine. Outwardly, I smirked at his sweaty face as he huffed and puffed, but deep down I was thankful. The fire of ambition was back in his eyes. His running gradually improved, and the treadmill became a friend not a foe. He started running outside, stepping into his new running gear to head out the door. Soon, "I have to run first" became a familiar phrase to our friends and family. It was a euphoria I was not privy to, no matter how he would try to explain it. It was freedom. The doctor agreed, and saw no need to continue his antidepressants.

On the work front we received the news that Michael had been one of the few applicants selected for a government-sponsored apprenticeship program. It allowed him to be paid weekly while going to school for retraining. In celebration, he signed up for his first 5K race; it became a new addiction. He wanted to run a marathon. It was a lofty goal, as the 5K run was painful and slow, but his mind was set. We became regular faces on the running circuit as he built his endurance on smaller runs. A small collection of finisher medals and bib numbers were hanging in our home. Our conversations were peppered with technical running terms and training regimes. I didn't mind any of it. His smile was back.

The day of his first marathon arrived. If I could only explain to you the electricity you feel when you stand among competing runners on race day. It hums in the air as you watch people engaging in their pre-race rituals. Michael was shaking his legs with nervous energy, constantly checking his watch while we waited for my in-laws and his sisters to show up. We walked around holding hands; we were happier now than ever. Over the course of the year we managed to move into a new home and get pregnant. I was seven months along.

The family clan arrived and we all stood at the starting gate and saw him off. We sat on the bleachers and waited, taking turns getting coffee, cheering on the runners. At the three-hour mark, we left the bleachers and weaved among the crowd to the finish line. Poised with our cameras, we fidgeted. Like a mirage, I finally spotted him in the distance running at a slow clip, his face in anguish. He had a slight limp. Relief flooded me as we cheered him on. He spotted us as he stumbled through the finishing gate. Corralled by race volunteers he was given water and ushered forward into the runner's pen.

It seemed like eternity, while I fought through the masses of people to see him on the other side. He had done it. I was so proud. He found us and waved. I ran forward as he opened his arms, and reached for me over the half fence. Tears streamed down his face and mine, and he began sobbing. "I love you. I could never have done this without you," he whispered in my ear through the tears.

Three weeks later we had a baby girl. To celebrate he decided to start training for his first triathlon.

~Carla O'Brien

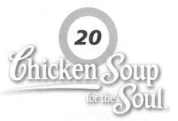

20

How Motherhood Made Me a Better Runner and Vice Versa

Running makes you an athlete in all areas of life... trained in the basics, prepared for whatever comes, ready to fill each hour and deal with the decisive moment.

~Dr. George Sheehan

I started running more than thirteen years ago as a form of stress relief while in my first year of law school. Never athletic growing up, I had always assumed myself to be doomed to a life of mediocrity when it came to anything remotely physical. Shortly after I took up running, though, my sister asked me to come run in a 5K fundraiser at the school where she was student teaching. Since I easily ran three to four miles each morning, I figured why not, especially since it was for a good cause. To my surprise, I won my age group, probably due in large part to the fact that most of the runners were students or parents and were not in my age group at the time. But that didn't matter to me—gift certificate and medal in hand, I was hooked.

Over the next seven years, I progressively competed in longer and longer distance races, eventually running my first marathon in 2000. I qualified for Boston on my first try and realized that I had, despite my poor athletic start to life, found something I could actually excel at. I got caught up in competing and, as a result, asked my dear husband, who was ready to start a family, to wait until I had gotten the competition "bug" out of my system before trying to have our first child.

The bug was finally satiated after I won the gold medal in the half marathon at the 2003 Pan-American Maccabi Games in Santiago, Chile. To me, that was the pinnacle of my running career to date and sufficient to finally take a rest from running competitively to give conceiving a child a shot. Little did I know that it would then take us two years and six rounds of in vitro fertilization (IVF) to actually accomplish that goal.

When we were going through the IVF cycles, I had to focus on daily injections and monitoring at the doctors' offices instead of running. After each negative pregnancy test and during the imposed rest month in between each IVF cycle, running was my only solace and sense of some return to normalcy from the emotional turmoil of infertility. Again, like in law school, it became my escape and form of stress relief.

We finally had success after traveling out of state to New York City to do one last cycle at a top fertility clinic. Running took a back seat when we found out we were expecting twins and I dared not do anything physical that could possibly jeopardize the long-desired pregnancy. For me to give up running for eight months was like a drug addict giving up cocaine, but it was an easy choice after all we had gone through to get pregnant.

Our twins were born in March 2006 and despite the exhaustion and haze of the first few months with twins, I returned to running to race my first 10K race just ten weeks after they were born. I ran my first postpartum marathon, alongside my husband, seven months later. Running then became my break from the constant needs of newborn twins. Thanks to a supportive husband who took on twin duty while I was working out or racing, I continued to train and compete for the next year and looked forward to returning to the Boston Marathon in April 2007. I even decided to do my first triathlon, something I had always wanted to do, in August of that year.

Those plans changed when I found out that we were unexpectedly (and spontaneously) pregnant with our third child just four weeks before the Boston Marathon. Again, running had to take a back seat for a few months. While it was frustrating to give up the opportunity to compete at Boston and in my first triathlon, I wasn't complaining after the difficulties we had conceiving our first children. Now we'd have three under the age of two.

After our third child was born in November 2007 I again returned to running and Boston and the triathlon were there waiting for me in 2008. Not only did I return to running and enter the world of triathlon, but somehow I did it at a level above where I had been performing when I was younger and before I had children, winning my age group and setting PRs in practically every road race and triathlon I entered. It didn't make sense to me: shouldn't I have been getting slower as I got older and had more children, hence less time?

I think several factors have made me a better athlete since I have had children: first, my time to train is so limited right now that I tend to focus much more and as a result get quality, instead of quantity, out of each training session. More importantly, though, the inspiration my children have provided me pushes me each and every race, even if they are not there in person. Setting a good example for my children is now my main source of motivation, not putting in more training hours than my competition or beating them in a race. It also doesn't hurt that my post-child training runs sometimes involve pushing 100 pounds of double stroller and children!

Not only has motherhood made me a better runner, but more importantly running has made me a better mother. It's not easy fitting in training and staying committed when trying to raise three young children, and there is always guilt when I take time away from them to train if I can't manage to fit it in before they wake up in the morning or after they go to bed. But I am learning to get over that guilt because after I get back from a run, a bike ride or a swim, my mind is clear, energy high, and I am a better mother than I would be if I didn't take that time for myself. Plus, excelling at something like running and triathlon has given me a confidence that has made me more secure with my decisions as a mother and, I hope, sets an example for my children.

Our kids have already run in their first organized fun runs, earned their finishers medals, and worn race numbers on their shirts. Our younger daughter's first words when she sees me in the morning are "Mommy sweaty?" since I usually greet them after returning from a pre-dawn workout. When they see a runner out on the roads they always say "a runner, like Mommy runs!" They tell me that one day they are going to be big and run as fast as Mommy. I hope they run even faster.

~Lisa Levin Reichmann

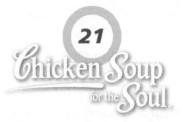

I'd Only Just Begun

Running the marathon gave me an inner strength that changed my life...
just finishing can have a profound effect on your confidence and self-esteem.
~Henley Gibble

I never thought I'd run a marathon. Then again, I never thought I'd get a divorce. It just so happened that in my case, for whatever reason, there seemed to be a fine thread that wove these two events together in my life.

I'd been a runner since high school. Never far. Never fast. Just consistent. Two or three miles a day, five or six times a week.

Marathons had always been unfathomable to me. How any human could run 26.2 miles was as foreign to me as swimming the English Channel or climbing Mount Everest. And when I realized that the best marathoners actually complete the trek in a little more than two hours, the only plausible explanation seemed that their bodies were created differently than mine.

The most essential ingredient to their success never occurred to me until the day a co-worker passed along a training schedule she had received from a friend. I glanced at it, chuckled and tossed it on top of a pile of things on my desk. But it was too late. The seed was planted.

There it was staring me in the face. Black and white instructions for making the impossible a reality. Sixteen weeks of training. Six days a week. Building up the mileage until some miracle transpired by week 14 and the long run actually broke 20 miles. As is the case so often in life, it all boiled down to one thing. Discipline.

The idea twirled around in my brain until one spring Saturday I took the matter out on the road to let my legs decide. Never before had I tried to run long. What if I kept going until I dropped? Maybe I'd be surprised at how far I could run.

Or not. Seven miles later, I stopped dead in my tracks, a mere 19.2 miles short. No matter. I was hooked.

An October marathon required my training to begin in June. It didn't take long to realize that I was never going to make it if I didn't find time for myself, an alien concept to me during those dark days. But suddenly I had a mission to accomplish. I would have to put work aside, find a sitter for my son and, quite literally, hit the road.

Six days a week, mile after mile after mile, I was alone with my thoughts. At a time when it seemed my entire life was collapsing around me, I was building something new. When it seemed as though everyone I ever trusted had let me down, I was learning to rely on myself. Even in the worst of moments, I discovered I could put on my Nikes and work it out on the road.

I ran past it all. The white lace and promises. The heavy anchor of expectations. The long shadow of religious obligation. Through it all, I kept running and running and running.

With every mile, I was getting stronger. I was gaining confidence. I was becoming reacquainted with the girl I had left behind somewhere. An impossible goal had been set and there was only one person who could make it happen.

Finally, the big day arrived. Even though my longest training run had barely broken 20 miles, there I was, poised in my new T-shirt on a warm October Sunday.

At the opening gun, I was buoyed along by the camaraderie of the event. The thousands of runners. The colorful shirts. The new running shoes. The theme song from *Rocky*. The exuberant crowd that lined the streets. I could run forever. I believed this. After ten miles, I still believed it. After eleven. After twelve.

But that would change.

After climbing a gut-wrenching hill, there was one neighborhood left to pass through before we would head for a long loop near the ocean. That's where it happened. I'd been warned it would come at around mile 20 or so. But at mile 14, there it was. The wall. Never in my life had I felt so defeated.

Whose crazy idea was this, anyway? Twenty-six miles. Why not a hundred? Why not a thousand? My feet stopped running. I started to walk. *This is the worst thing you've ever tried to do. Who are you kidding? You'll never make it.* I couldn't go on.

Then a man came out of the crowd and stood alongside me. He didn't say a word. He didn't ask what was wrong. He just smiled and started to walk with me. Despite my despair, I found myself matching my stride to his, just as I had so many times before.

A half mile later, I was ready to run again. I asked my dad why he'd chosen that particular spot to watch for me. He just hugged me and said he'd be waiting at the finish line.

And finish, I did.

I still remember it all. The foil cape wrapped around my shoulders to keep the heat in. The shiny medal around my neck. Not because I won. But because I had actually done it. I remember the hugs and the handshakes, too. How they came at me from every direction. A surreal moment for a lifetime.

I should have been ecstatic. But I was content to sit and drink a bottle of water. I had accomplished what once, for me, had seemed impossible. I had made it from start to finish. From there to here.

As it turned out, my marriage ended with far less fanfare. The final papers arrived amid a pile of junk mail on a gray winter's day. An official proclamation that someone I had relied on for so long wasn't going to be there anymore. But by the time it came, I was ready. Because I'd learned to rely on someone else.

Myself.

~Rita Lussier

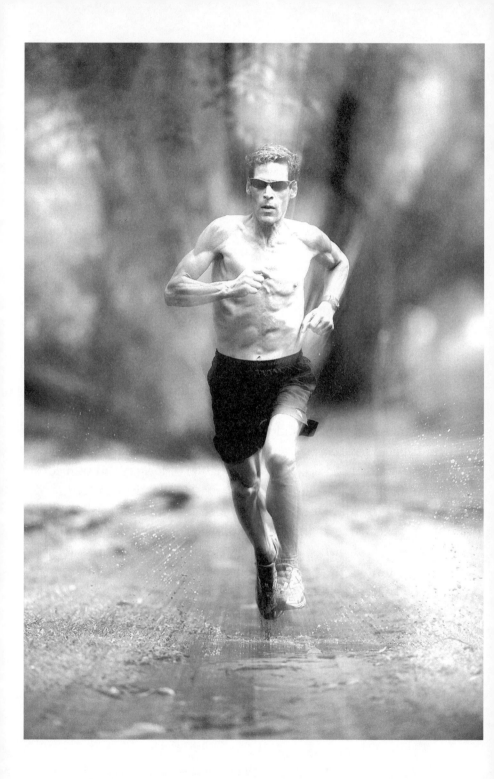

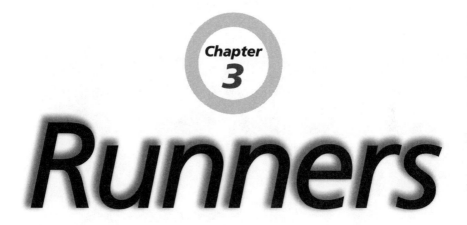

Chapter 3

Runners

Camaraderie

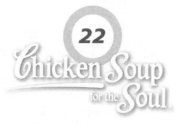

22

The Kindness of Runners

Winning has always meant much to me,
but winning friends has meant the most.
~Babe Zaharias

Every so often, something happens that reminds you just how great our sport is. One of those somethings happened for me on a quiet summer morning in upstate New York.

My wife and I were away for a long weekend, celebrating our first wedding anniversary at an old, sprawling Shawangunk Mountain resort. It was a beautiful place—a very oak-paneled-lobby, open-lake-swim, Sunday-lobster-bake, porches-and-rocking-chairs sort of hideaway.

Think *The Shining*, but with less blood in the halls and more croquet.

Thing was, I was training for a fall marathon at the time. So, beauty aside, I was a little anxious about the 14-miler I had planned for Sunday. Not about being able to run 14 miles, but about being able to do so on such unfamiliar turf. We were surrounded by "2,200 acres of scenic wilderness," according to the booklet in our room, including 85 miles of trails. But I'd been having trouble keeping my bearings on them. (Hey, 85 miles of trails was about 71 miles more than I needed.) Doing an easy 4-mile loop was no problem, even for someone as navigationally challenged as me. Four miles, I could handle. But I was fairly certain I'd get lost and die trying to navigate a 14-mile run out there. The phrase "skeletal remains" leapt to mind.

But you've gotta do what you've gotta do, so I set out early

Sunday morning with my wristband I.D. and a bottle of orange Gatorade from the gift shop. The sun was shining, which was nice. If I was going to get lost and die, at least it would happen in agreeable weather.

The first few miles rolled by reasonably well, despite a dead end and some backtracking. Then I saw them: A group of six or eight fellow runners, on the same trail, headed right for me.

As we neared each other, we exchanged the usual nods and greetings. Then I stopped. Feeling a little sheepish, I asked, "Umm... How far are you guys going?"

"20," one of them said. "We just started."

Even more sheepish: "You mind if I... uh... join you for part of it?"

"Sure."

So I did. Off we went. And what followed were 10 of the nicest miles I think I've ever run.

Time flew by, and my newfound friends—all locals—knew the trails backward and front. The scenery, all ponds and pine and postcard vistas, was breathtaking. Even the pace was just right. We chatted here and there, as they told me a bit about the trails and the local running scene and themselves. They asked about me and my wife, my work and my running, so we talked about those things too.

Four of them were training for that fall's New York City Marathon. A couple had run the Richmond Marathon, the race I was training for. (They gave me some pointers about the course.) One guy had run sub-3 hours at Boston a few months prior. A woman had started with the elites another year, also at Boston, which is pretty hard-core. They were active members of a local running club. Several of them were teachers. All of them were funny and thoughtful.

Just like that, my morning run had gone from "solo wander" to "group run." And it was so seamless, happening so quickly, without question or fanfare. It all unfolded so... *naturally*. It almost didn't occur to me to stop and appreciate how very cool it was.

But I did appreciate it, both during the run and afterward. That's the thought that's really stuck with me, to this very day: *How great is our sport, where you can stumble across a group of strangers running in the middle of nowhere, and join them as if it's the most natural thing in the world?*

In a society more and more splintered, and drawn more and more to virtual, online "community," it's such a privilege to be part of a warm, far-reaching, real-life community. It's just one of many, many things to love about running. But it's one of the most satisfying things.

I know from talking with other runners that mine isn't an isolated story. When you're a runner in an unfamiliar place, very rarely are you ever truly alone, unless you want to be. Head out the door of your hotel in just about any city or town, and it's fairly likely you'll encounter a fellow runner or three at some point. (To paraphrase Yogi Berra: Wherever runners go, there you are.) And they'll probably welcome a bit of company, if you ask. You're a runner, after all. You must be a decent person. C'mon. Let's run.

It's a phenomenon I call "The Kindness of Runners," and it cuts across social, racial, economic, and geographic lines. It's a pretty marvelous thing.

• • •

Just shy of 2 hours into my own run, our group came to a fork in the trail. The locals told me they were going left, to finish their 20-miler; I should turn right, which would get me back to the resort at just around 14 miles.

I thanked them. They replied, "you bet" and "no problem" and "have a good one." As I ran off, one of them turned to call out, "Happy anniversary!"

Then they rounded a bend, and vanished from sight.

• • •

Later that same year, I would bump into two of my Shawangunk trail buddies at the New York City Marathon expo. I was there selling and signing copies of my new book. They were there because they were running the race. I'll admit, when they first approached me in my booth, I didn't recognize them—they were wearing jeans and jackets, after all, not shorts and technical tees. And it had been months since our run together in the mountains. Besides which, the New York City Marathon expo is a dizzying place, teeming with foot traffic; you're lucky to recognize your own mother in a crowd like that.

Still, as they shook my hand and reintroduced themselves, it all came back in a flash. Shawangunk! My best 14-miler ever! Yes! Hey, how *are* you?

We chatted for a minute or so, then more hand-shaking and well-wishing. Then they rejoined the swarm and I got back to hawking books.

The memories lingered, though. I couldn't stop thinking back to that trail run in August, to the brilliant sunshine and the stunning views. More than anything, I recalled the companionship and camaraderie, and the warmth I felt—not from the sun, but simply from being out there, running. With some new friends.

~Mark Remy

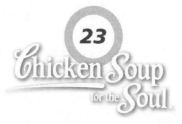

23

The Pre-Dawn People

I'd like mornings better if they started later.
~Author Unknown

t just after 4 AM, the alarm went off and I reached over and contemplated my life choices as I fumbled awkwardly to shut off the annoying buzzing before it awoke my sleeping spouse. He heard me anyway.

"Why are you getting up so early?" he said in a highbrow tone that suggested early risers were at the bottom of the totem pole of polite society.

"I have to interview those runners," I sighed as I heaved myself from the bed. I winced as my first warm foot touched the icy floor. Was the money worth this?

"Who gets up at this hour to exercise?" he mumbled as he rolled over in our previously shared nest of toasty marital bliss.

Who, indeed? I looked over my shoulder and considered ditching the interview. It was the perfect opportunity to get two hours of the exceptional sleep one experiences only when dodging an adult responsibility.

I'd taken a freelance writing job to cover a group of runners who I decided must be crazy to rise so early just to exercise. Didn't they realize some gyms are open 24 hours? Why the hurry? What sort of drive must it take to slither from warm blankets and tread outside so early in the morning?

I used to be a runner. As I poured my coffee I tried to remember my sleek thighs and toned arms, back in the days when I started every morning with a brisk run. That was pre-husband and pre-teenagers. Between working, a family, and housework, I was lucky to get to bed before midnight. But here I was, about to interview a group of pre-dawn people with almost supernatural motivation.

I could understand if work beckoned them so early from the comfort of their beds. But it was exercise!

When I jumped into my car and drove off, I thought about the runners. I wondered what type of people I would find at the dough-nut shop's parking lot, where the runners began their daily routine. Did they work? They couldn't possibly have kids or real responsibilities, right?

Surely there wouldn't be many people to interview. It was dark, cold, and foggy. I pulled into the empty parking lot and shut off my car's engine, instantly feeling the chill creep in through the floor-board. I wanted to go home.

I'm glad I didn't leave. My life was about to change.

One by one, sets of headlights turned into the deserted parking lot — because inside the cars were people who'd been running together before dawn for decades, and they knew they would be held accountable if they didn't show up. They arrived smiling; I was mystified.

I got out of my car and joined a group that was heading toward the doughnut shop. For thirteen years, the runners had been using the doughnut shop as home base, but the group had been around much longer than that. It had been going strong for forty years.

Forty years of running together? What was I missing? I looked around. The air was crisp, the coffee was hot, and camaraderie was in abundance. Was that it?

Coffee wasn't what motivated dozens of runners to show up every day before dawn. As I chatted with two women, I learned that most started to maintain physical fitness, but even the health benefits of running had become a secondary motivation for setting alarm clocks so early.

No one looked as grouchy as I felt. None of them appeared sleep deprived. In fact, just the opposite was true. They were peppy!

After making initial contact, I backed off to observe — more from genuine curiosity (and a bit of envy) than for the article I was writing. I wanted to figure out why they were so happy, why they seemed like a big, functional family.

Slowly, they began breaking off into groups. Some ran with a dog, but all ran with a smile.

No one ran with an iPod. Conversation provided the musical cadence to which these runners ran. I found out that the running becomes a sort of counseling session for them as they talk and solve the world's problems. They share stories about life, routine day to day things, tragedy, experiencing 9/11 together, loss, and laughter.

The more they shared with me, the more I was beginning to understand the force that would pull them from bed each day. They didn't mind the alarm clock because to them, it wasn't exercise — it was recreation.

One runner looked pointedly at me and asked, "Why don't you join us?"

"Oh, no, I couldn't," I said quickly, and then wondered why I couldn't. I was standing among busy mothers of toddlers and white-collar executives, who still had to drive home to shower so they could get to the office by 8:00. How was my situation unique? My responsibilities were no more time-consuming than theirs.

I was missing out, and I was realizing that my physical health wasn't the only loser in the scenario.

Most of the runners had met through their mutual love of the sport, and many of them had booked "running vacations" together, had camped with each other, and had celebrated holidays as a group. They'd nursed one another through illness, death, family crisis, and job loss, but they'd celebrated births and marriages, too.

I learned that one runner had lost his first wife — another runner — in a tragic accident. Years later, when he was ready to marry again, the group attended his wedding — on the trail. One hundred runners ran two miles up a steep hill and surrounded him with love. The loss of his wife was hard for the whole team, but they were overjoyed to see him happy again.

After hearing the story, I stood in stunned silence as my heart swelled with pride in the human spirit. Someone came up behind me. She was another runner, and she'd overheard my last conversation.

"I think people initially show up so they have someone to run with, someone to push them," she said as she toweled off her face. "Somewhere along the miles, though, it shifts. We show up because our friends are here."

That's when it clicked for me. In other words, it's about fitness and friendship, and to runners who've chosen to exercise as a group, you can't have one without the other.

I collected enough information for my story that day, wrote the article, and was paid. But the value I received at the doughnut shop far outweighed the compensation that the magazine gave me for the article.

I wish I could say that I awoke bright and early the next day and began running with the group, but I can't. I still enjoy sleeping until 6:00. However, my life did change. The runners taught me that happiness comes from being fit, living right, and building healthy relationships.

I did start running again, and I am running to this day.

I don't get up at 4 AM, but the road doesn't care. The road is glad to see me any time of day.

~Dana Martin

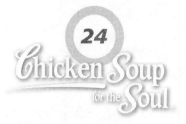

24

I Am a Hasher

*Do not go where the path may lead, go instead where there is no path
and leave a trail.*
~Ralph Waldo Emerson

I have a confession, I am a hasher. No, that doesn't mean I smoke weed. "Hasher" is what members of the "Hash House Harrier" running group call themselves.

A name steeped in wartime history for British expats, these "drinkers with a running problem" simply were out to get some exercise, rid themselves of the weekend excess and celebrate their good living with a cold one. The housing complex in which they lived was called the "Hash House," and the game they played was "Hares and Hounds." When the Malaysian government required the group to register with a name back in 1938, the Hash House Harriers was simple enough.

After World War II, the remaining members split up and went home. Having enjoyed the camaraderie of their runs in Kuala Lumpur, each started his own chapters of the original, eventually causing the group to grow worldwide.

However, this is not a history lesson. It's the start of what—for me—was a world adventure, and one particular group which gave me an everlasting memory of what it is to belong.

I was born and raised in Las Vegas. Which, contrary to popular belief, doesn't fly its populace in from California. It was here that I started hashing, brought in on a whim by a cute girl with a crazy

T-shirt and a business card that had the group hotline number on the back.

Not knowing what to expect, I called the number later that night and listened to a pre-recorded message with directions to the local wetlands preserve and advising me to bring a flashlight, a whistle and a thirst for the "golden nectar" (which I thankfully learned later was beer).

I ran cross country in high school, but never at twilight, and while we had water, I was at the time clueless to what golden nectar could refer to.

Dialing my brother, I described the message to him and asked if he would join me in attending this trail run, what with me not knowing anyone else there. He told me it sounded like a cult and then hung up.

Well, I've always thought there was nothing to lose by going out on the limb, except for a little face, so I put on my shoes and drove down to the starting point.

As I pulled into the parking area, I found the most motley group of individuals. With my matching name-brand running shirt, shorts and shoes, I must have stood out like a sore thumb. Here people were drinking beer while dressed in Day-Glo shirts with the sleeves ripped off, multi-color headbands, mismatched socks and shoes that looked like they'd endured the Trail of Tears.

One man came up to me, introduced himself as "Reverend Right Hand" and pointed out a few others to me with insane names like "Hunka Hunka" and "Blueberry Hill-less" along with some names that would make my grandmother blush.

Everyone stood in a circle and they took an empty beer bottle and spun it in the center of the group. It landed on one gentleman who took a large bag filled with flour and started running, leaving large dollops on the ground behind him. Right Hand told me to wait a couple of minutes and they did the silliest warm-up exercise I've ever seen before we took off as a pack and chased down the man with the flour.

Catching up to him first, he thrust the bag in my hand, pointed me in a direction and said, "Go, you've got a three-minute head start!"

I stood there with a blank look and told him that I hadn't a clue what to do. He replied, "Run, and don't forget to leave flour behind you! You've got 2 minutes and 45 seconds!"

And that was it. I bolted into the reeds, frantically dropping flour behind me. There was a hiking path through the wetlands but I don't really remember using much of it. What I do remember is the thrill of being chased, the freedom of creating my own path and the exhilaration of hearing a dozen whistles blowing with yells of "On-On!" from the other side of a large thicket. Eventually someone caught up to me and I was relieved of my flour burden, once again the hound and not the hare. I was hooked.

In the past five years I have run with over 100 different hashes, logged in over 1,000 miles, worn about 10 pairs of shoes through the sole and loved every minute of it. Being a hasher may be the best part of my life. The group is more a brotherhood and it doesn't take much to experience its hash-pitality.

I took a year to travel around the world and nine times out of ten, I had a place to stay. I'd arrive in a foreign country and a hasher would meet me at the train station, take me out for a drink and give me a couch for the night, simply because another hasher had called to say I was coming.

And the running was gorgeous! As a tourist you see what tourists see. As a hasher you get to experience the real country through the eyes of a runner. Forested hills in Switzerland, ancient castle ruins in Germany and Scotland, rice fields in Thailand, rural villages in Cambodia, the barrios of the Philippines. Then later you drink local beer in local bars, surrounded by people who may not always speak your language, but understand the language of a good drink. It was the time of my life and one I'll never forget. It showed me that a great winding trail and a willingness to imbibe in the ridiculousness of our zest for adventure in a pair of shoes isn't limited to a wetlands park in Las Vegas, but is shared around the world.

~Jeff Hoyt, AKA Alcoholiday,
Las Vegas Hash House Harriers

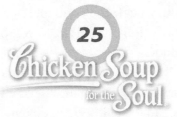

25

That Should Have Been a Left

I have never been lost, but I will admit to being confused for several weeks.
~Daniel Boone

Individually and in small groups of two and three, runners stumbled like survivors of a shipwreck toward their cars. Dripping sweat, they poured water down parched throats. Few things in life compare to running in North Carolina humidity. In mid-summer, the air is thick enough to hold a mosquito mid-flight. But more than just hot, the runners were discouraged. For the fifth time in as many weeks, the cue sheet for the group run had been wrong, tacking on an additional 1.95 miles to an already miserable 15-mile run.

"Sorry guys," said Marisa, our running coach. She had the decency to look embarrassed. "That right turn onto Cotswold listed on the cue sheet? That should have been a left."

We let her live only because we were too whipped as a group to summon the energy required to knock her down.

This was year two of a marathon-training program. The first year, the owners of a specialty running store in town had run the program, preparing many of us for what would be our first marathon. Having caught the running bug, most of our group had returned for another season. With the popularity of the training program growing, the store owners hired a professional trainer to take over the daily logistics of transforming a group of so-so runners into marathon-ready competitors.

Our trainer Marisa is a 5'10" brunette beauty with a soft voice and an absent-mindedness more readily associated with blondes. But behind the girly veneer beats the heart of a warrior. While training our group, Marisa was preparing for her third Ironman competition. Which made us wonder, as we complained about having to do speed work or run yet another 10-miler, if she on some occasions just wanted to smack us. The feeling, however, was often reciprocal.

"I can't believe the cue sheet was wrong again," moaned one runner. "How hard is it to map a route?"

"Doesn't she drive the route she plans for us?" said another runner, pouring water over her head. "I'm tired of getting lost."

She had a point. On the tangled streets of Greensboro, North Carolina, pockets of us running at different paces criss-crossed one another's paths as we tried to decipher where exactly, this time, the cue sheet had gone wrong.

"We've already passed this park twice."

"Let's backtrack to the last traffic light and try going straight."

"I swear to God, I'm quitting and calling my wife to come get me if we don't figure this out in the next mile."

For her part, Marisa seemed oblivious to how disheartening it was for our group to mentally prepare for a 14-mile run and then be forced to run 17 due to cue sheet malfunctions.

"Just think how strong you're getting!" she chirped.

We didn't feel strong. We hurt. Marisa's training didn't resemble what we'd done the year before. That first year, our group mainly met just to run. This year, Marisa introduced us to ab work, fartleks, hills that rivaled what a person seeking to climb Mount Everest might do, and a particularly evil concept known as a "progression" run where we were told to pick up speed throughout the run, ending with an all-out sprint.

But over the course of three months, something miraculous happened. Our times improved. Hills that once reduced us to tears now weren't so hard. And getting lost every Sunday on our long run became less of a misery and more of a standing joke.

"Here are the cue sheets," said Marisa, passing out the thin slips of paper late in the season. "Today's run is 19 miles."

"That means 30!" cried the group, winking and nudging each other.

"No, no. Seriously, I triple checked this," said Marisa, her face earnest. "This one is 19."

When we stumbled in at 20.2 with yet another left missing from the sheet, Marisa held her head in her hands. "I'm so sorry!" she exclaimed. "I went over and over that sheet. I can't believe I missed that."

Finally, our race days arrived. We e-mailed each other good luck and followed the split times of runners through online race sites. Again and again, runners from our group met or exceeded their goals. "I felt strong," more than one person e-mailed the group about their finish.

Marisa is training next year's group and all of us are eager to re-enlist. Like the pain of a marathon, the sting of an erroneous cue sheet quickly fades from the mind. If anything, those long, hot summer runs where we stumbled lost through the streets brought us together as a group. So much so, that we decided to purchase T-shirts to commemorate our time spent together.

The white wicking shirts are a tribute to simplicity. On the front, they have the name given to our group by Marisa, "Team Evolve." And on the back, in block letters, one short phrase that will forever bring a smile to the lips of every runner in our group from that summer.

"That Should Have Been A Left."

~Dena Harris

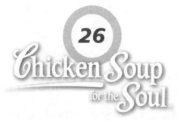

Cross Country Isn't for Wimps

My sport is your sport's punishment.
~Anonymous

Let's be honest. When you think of the cross country athlete, the term "tough guy" isn't exactly the first thing to jump into your mind.

There are no bone-jarring collisions and no broken bones. Runners can be sidelined by a hangnail or a sore toe. They can be knocked out of action by a head cold, a bee sting or a bout with hay fever.

Runners don't even talk much trash, and you never hear of a race being suspended because of a brawl.

Truth be told, cross country is a sport inhabited by tall, skinny people like me, most of whom wouldn't survive a fraction of the physical abuse that occurs on the gridiron.

But that doesn't mean cross country is a sport for wimps. Far from it.

Perhaps what makes cross country such a tough sport is the price it exacts from its athletes. There's no resting, no taking a play off or relying on your teammates to pick up your slack.

Stand at a finish line and you'll understand what I mean. Finishers rarely stride across the line. They wash over it like driftwood, completely emptied of all energy and will. Some stumble and some collapse. Some are carried out by race officials.

This is not a sport for wimps.

This is a sport for the stout of heart. This is a sport for those who are willing to discover the limits of their endurance and then push themselves beyond it, knowing that the runners panting just behind them are prepared to do the same.

Several years ago, I witnessed an odd delay while watching the California High School Cross Country Finals at Woodward Park in Fresco, CA. The Division I runners were left to mill around the starting line nervously, stretching and taking practice sprints while they waited for the signal to take their marks.

Finally, the event announcer explained the cause of the delay. The final Division V runner was still on the course, and Division I couldn't start until he got out of their way.

"Just now finishing," I thought. "At the 33:00 mark?"

As he made his way around the final bend and up toward the finish, a smattering of applause arose from the athletes at the starting line.

What a sight it was. Straddling the starting line were some of the fastest cross country runners in California, mere seconds from the biggest race of their lives. Several yards away was this poor kid, holding up the action as he struggled to complete his race a full 8 minutes behind his nearest competitor.

And the Division I runners were cheering him on.

I didn't understand at the moment why they were doing it, so I chalked it up to good sportsmanship. It wasn't until after I'd watched several hundred other runners wash over the finish line that I grasped what the ovation was all about.

It was a show of respect.

Runners understand how demanding cross country can be. Hundreds of hours of training. Cramps, nausea, vomiting, burning lungs, blurred vision, and wobbling legs.

They recognize that anyone with the guts to go through what it takes to compete at any level deserves respect, regardless of how fast he runs. Not that they demand respect for themselves. They don't.

But they do give it freely to those who run alongside them.

That's the unique camaraderie of cross country. It's the camaraderie that comes from sharing the same foxhole.

~Bob Dickson

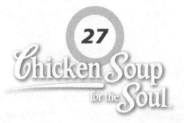

Running Blind

What a blind person needs is not a teacher but another self.
~Helen Keller

O ur story began when I responded to a blind runner's request on the local runners club website. He asked if anyone would be interested in volunteering to be his sighted running guide.

"Ha," said one of my daughters. "That would be the blind leading the blind."

She wasn't necessarily referring to my eyesight with her remark. It's more about how I'm not the most coordinated athlete on the street. In fact, I was once politely asked to not jog on the club's treadmill since my predilection for getting tossed off, going airborne and then crash landing into the yoga classroom was considered disruptive to the others.

I hate treadmills as much as they apparently hate me and so I took to the open road, lonely paths and happy trails.

I wasn't the most qualified person to guide a blind runner but as it turned out, I was the only one who replied to his e-mail.

Before our first outing, I asked my smart-aleck daughter to practice with me. Somehow, I convinced her to wear a blindfold and let me guide her down the street.

I yelled "curb!" just as she tumbled head first into the garbage cans.

"That went well," I said, hopefully, as she threw off the blindfold and declared me unfit for service.

I did a little research before we met. He was a perfectly sighted police office, writing a routine traffic ticket, when a drunk driver crashed her car into him. His head slammed onto the cruiser and, multiple brain surgeries later, he emerged from near death with scars, crushed bones and a completely pulverized optic nerve.

Before his injury, he was a runner who loved nothing more than to run outside. Since his recovery, he'd been condemned to running on a treadmill, something he despised as much as I did.

Using adaptive software to communicate by e-mail and text message, I got directions to his house and picked him up early one morning. He showed me how we'd run "tethered" with a shoelace held in my right hand and his left hand.

We started off with a slow trot, my heart pounding as loud as his shoes clomping next to me. He was double my weight and height and his stride was at least double mine. I scurried like a little rat to keep up with him. It was a balmy day, not a cloud in the sky and a few runners headed our way.

"Hey, what do I do about, uh, here comes some runners," I say to him. I started to get anxious.

The runners were coming straight for us and there wasn't any way I could move his bulk far enough to the side of the path, without him toppling over.

Frantically, I waved at the runners, motioning them to pass me on the left.

In exchange, I got what would become a typical reaction.

Annoyance, irritation and the occasional middle finger as we hogged the path instead of passing single file like considerate runners.

Eventually, the other runners must have figured it out because they began saying hello as they passed, waving at me ahead of time and generally scooting out of the way.

We have some rules when we run. If we start to sink into negative commentary, we change the channel immediately. Of course, he has a lot more to be negative about than just about anyone I know but we don't dwell on that. Instead, we use the time to really look at the world.

I start off every run by describing the weather. He wants to know about the clouds, the wind and the sun. As we trot along, I give him his bearings. The river is on the left, a barge is coming from the south, a hawk is flying overhead, I tell him as our foot strikes synch up.

Before I was a sighted guide, I ran blindly through the miles. Instead of listening to birds or the rhythm of my feet on the path, I blasted the Rolling Stones into my headphones, muting nature with the flick of a finger. The part of me not absorbed by the music calculated the miles, marking them off like a dreaded to-do list. Only 2.5 miles left to go, I'd tell myself, trying to cajole my reluctant feet.

All that changed when I became his eyes. Suddenly, I had to really be present. I had to focus intently on the moment, scouring the path for obstacles. A branch blown onto the path by a gust of wind could trip him face first into the gravel.

Once, we were engrossed in a conversation about the best running songs when I couldn't get my brain around what was draped across the trail. I would have screamed but my vocal chords froze. Somehow, our feet sailed in unison across the sunning copperhead and it wasn't until he was singing the chords of "Born to Run" that I fell completely apart.

"Snake!" I yelled, weak with relief.

He told me later that his legs turned to spaghetti.

It hit him full force that he was completely dependent on me. On my skills, my powers, my sense of direction. My ability.

"Yeah, that must be more scary than a snake," said my daughter, shaking her head.

It is. Or it was.

But over time, he's developed a sense of trust that gives me a sense of purpose. I run with new confidence and heightened senses. I anticipate obstacles before they even arrive.

Over the miles of stories we tell, some common themes emerge. His utter devotion to his wife and unborn son top the list. She's permanently seared in his memory and will never age past his last glimpse of her. We discuss current events, new books and Alabama football.

Mostly, we talk about things that go right in our lives. At some point, we argue over our choice for the best running song ever.

"We need a theme song. You know, something that sums up our running partnership," he says one day. I'm leery. I'm not a "what's your song," kind of gal. But he's humming as I trot alongside, waiting to see what he comes up with. Finally, he grins and says, "I got it!"

And then, as we sprint to the car, he sings "I can see clearly now, the rain is gone. I can see all the obstacles in the way."

"Here comes the sun," I tell my daughter later. She rolls her eyes.

"Did he notice you can't carry a tune in a bucket?"

He's never mentioned it.

~Carolyn Magner Mason

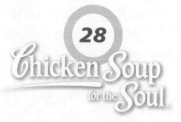

Trail and Error

The trail is the thing, not the end of the trail.
Travel too fast and you miss all you are traveling for.
~Louis L'Amour

"No one," announced an official with a clipboard, "has ever dropped out of this race."

I swallowed.

Three months ago, when I registered, it sounded romantic — the Superior Trail 25K, a 15.5-mile race on the Superior Hiking Trail. I pictured myself, sunlit and songbird-serenaded, bounding through the trees like the star of a shoe commercial.

Then I read the course description.

"The trail winds through boreal forests of birch, spruce, balsam fir and alder as it climbs to the top of Moose Mountain. A lot of ups and downs make this a very challenging section to run. This is one of the toughest sections of the Superior Hiking Trail and caution must be observed."

Now it was early on a May Saturday, on a dusty road in Lutsen. Start time was two minutes away.

A pine-scented breeze cooled my nervous sweat. Around me, the other runners stretched their quads, kissed their spouses, knotted their shoelaces, and pinned their race numbers to their shirts. Friends and relatives hovered on the edges of the crowd, snapping pictures, slapping high-fives and shouting good luck. I braced my hands on my hips and reminded myself to breathe. Despite my months of preparation, I felt like a student who forgot to study for a test. I had trained on roads.

Road running is about rhythms—fast music, steady breathing, staccato slap of soles on pavement. None of those rhythms would serve me on this trail. Roots, ravines, and lack of asphalt would preclude a consistent pace. "A lot of ups and downs" would make my breathing anything but steady. And the Superior Trail Race discourages headphone use because, as the website explains, "Full awareness of one's surroundings, and the ability to communicate with other participants, race volunteers, and trail users unassociated with the event are critical to everyone's safety."

The official counted down the final seconds. "Five, four, three…"

I swallowed again.

The horn blasted. I started running. Everything, I told myself, would be just fine. "Mountain" and "challenging" were relative terms.

A few miles into the race, on a long switchback section that had me sucking air like an asthmatic, I kicked myself for leaving my MP3 player at home. Music would distract me from my aching thighs and mud-soaked, squelching shoes. Rules be damned. I could have tucked the player in my pocket until I was out of sight of the officials. And the other entrants couldn't rat me out; for now, at least, there were none in sight.

A stitch worked its way up my left side. A nascent blister burned my right heel. Hunger torqued my gut like someone wringing out a rag. (I had been too anxious to eat breakfast.) A college friend's philosophy on racing got more appealing by the minute.

"It's against my morals," he always says. "I only run when chased."

Voices echoed up the trail. Laughter.

I glanced back and saw a pack of women coming up behind me. I debated whether to pick up my pace to stay ahead of them or slow down so they would pass me. It didn't even occur to me that I could run with them. I trained alone—why should a race be different?

The voices got closer. I slowed and moved right.

A dark-haired woman who looked to be in her forties passed me at an easy lope. She settled into her stride a few yards ahead of me.

"Hello," she called in an infuriatingly unlabored voice.

I gasped a reciprocal greeting and hoped she would leave it at that. Unlike her, I had no air to spare for conversation.

She glanced back and introduced herself. I managed to respond with my name and a windy "Nice to meet you."

"Do you want," she asked, "to run with my friends and me?"

I hesitated. I had trained alone, so I wasn't accustomed to running with people. I would feel humiliated if I couldn't keep up with them. But, then again, their presence might inspire me to push myself harder than solitude would. And this race was nothing like training.

"Sure."

She introduced me to the other women. Turns out they were veteran runners in their late fifties—I told them I had thought they were in their forties, and this conjured big smiles—with a dozen ultramarathons between them. The dark-haired one asked how old I was.

"I'm twenty."

She shook her head as if in dismay, but she was smiling. "I've been running," she said, "longer than you've been alive."

Keeping up was tough but worth it. We talked during the flat sections and huffed and puffed up the steep parts. At the aid station at the halfway point, I sucked down a salt pill, a handful of M&Ms, half a peanut butter sandwich and two Dixie cups of Coke. My stomach gurgled its appreciation.

Two of the women waited for me. "Ready?"

After the race, the dark-haired woman hugged me. "You did great," she said. "I'm proud of you."

This, I realized, was the key difference between road running and trail running. Connection. On the trail there was no asphalt between my feet and the earth, no headphones between my ears and the birdsongs, no distance between myself and the people around me.

~Shelby Gonzalez

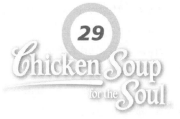

Who Is Robert DeVille?

The only competition of a wise man is with himself.
~Washington Allston

A few years back, a running buddy of mine we call Lucky Jim called me up on a Saturday night. He knew it was short notice, but he was in a bind. He and a group of his co-workers were entered in a team-only 10K the next morning. One of their runners was still out of town on company business and wouldn't be back in time for the race.

"Can you fill in for him?" he asked. "If we can't get a substitute we'll be disqualified and won't be able to run. The entry fee is paid, you get his T-shirt and there's food and a keg after."

"I don't know," I said. "You guys are pretty competitive. I'm not even close to being in your league time-wise."

"Doesn't matter," he said. "We just want to be able to run. Don't even worry about your time."

After some more cajoling, I finally agreed to meet them at the race site in the morning. It was going to be another beautiful fall day and I was planning on getting in a few miles anyway, so why not.

"Remember, your name is Robert DeVille," he said. "I doubt that anyone will ask, but if they do you're Robert DeVille."

"Robert DeVille. Got it," I replied.

After a brief introduction, my new "teammates," a group of ultra-fit, twenty-something guys and gals, were off and gone at the start, leaving me well behind to finish at my relaxed, plodding pace. When I met up with them at the beer tent, things weren't as mellow as I was led to believe. Evidently these folks were pretty serious about winning this event, or at least placing high. Most of their muffled conversation dealt with the fact that if the REAL Robert DeVille had been running instead of yours truly, that might have been a distinct possibility. From what I gathered as they distanced themselves from me was that this Robert DeVille was quite the stud.

Not that I cared. I had a few beers with Lucky Jim, and said my goodbyes, accepted a few chilly "thanks for filling in's" and was off. My life as Robert DeVille was over.

About six months later I was running in my first race of the new year, a 15K over a grueling, hilly course. I was on the homestretch, a flat mile and a half to the finish line. Suddenly everyone in front of me began splitting off to the left or right side of the road. There, dead center, was a downed runner, medical personnel already attending to him. He was out cold. I hoped he would be all right, and continued to the finish line.

At the refreshment tent I met up with Lucky Jim and a couple of other friends, who as per usual, had finished well ahead of me.

"Hey, did you guys see the guy who went down in the middle of the road back there?" I asked.

"Yeah!" said Lucky Jim. "I just talked to this girl we work with. She went and checked on him. He's going to be alright. I guess he hadn't been training much and he just came out too hard, especially on the hills. He just passed out."

"You know that guy?" I asked.

"Of course! You remember… oh wait! You've never met!"

"Not that I recall. Who is he?"

"Robert DeVille! That's Robert DeVille!"

~Lee Hammerschmidt

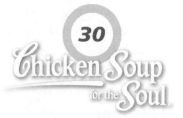

30

Running with Geezers

Age is not measured by years....
Some people are born old and tired while others are going strong at seventy.
~Dorothy Thompson

You've heard the phrase "Never judge a book by its cover?" Nowhere is this more true than in the world of marathon running. Men and women who—from appearances—look better suited to rocking chairs in front of nursing homes than running 26.2, blow by thirty-something hard bodies heaving by the side of the road. The lesson? Age is just a number—especially when it comes to running.

I run with geezers, men almost a quarter century older than me. This intrigues people who don't shy away from asking why I don't run with peers. Their faces betray their suspicion that I'm working toward some sort of merit badge, as if completing a 10-mile run with people allowed an AARP discount compares to helping the homeless or saving puppies. Very decent of me.

My morning running partners, Jack and Royce, are both in their sixties. We meet twice a week at 5:30 AM to run in our small North Carolina town. Royce's wife, a lovely woman with a terrific sense of humor, bears the brunt of small town teasing.

"Hey," say the tellers at our local bank, winking at one another as she walks in. "We've seen Royce running around town with another woman."

She doesn't miss a beat. "I know," she says. "And if I could catch her, I'd do something about it."

Why geezers? Friendships among runners blossom for many reasons, but the deepest bonds form among those who run the same pace. (I'm sure seven-minute milers are lovely people. Alas, I'm destined never to know them.) But what most non-runners fail to grasp is that age and pace aren't tied together. The perfect example of this comes from my friend Dave who has been running marathons and ultramarathons for almost forty years. Dave tells the story of his first running coach, a man fifteen years his senior. In their first marathon together, when Dave was nineteen and his coach thirty-four, the coach grabbed Dave at the start line and said, "Let's get something straight. You're younger than me and you're faster. You'll beat me in any 5K and in today's race you'll be ahead of me at mile 10 and maybe even mile 15. But son," and here the coach patted Dave on the back and gave a slow smile. "Just so you know. When we reach mile 20, your ass is mine."

I live that truth. Experience trumps my youth and enthusiasm every time. Even on short runs, my geezers maintain a steady stream of dialogue as I wheeze and gasp behind them. I may be twenty to thirty years younger than my running partners, but that simply means these guys have twenty to thirty years of training on me. "Respect the miles," they tell me, and I do.

True gentlemen, my geezers have never treated me as anything less than a running equal. When we run, we stride side by side. (Unless there's a car. Then, I inevitably find myself sandwiched, protected from ahead and behind. This never fails to both amuse and comfort me.) In the beginning, they patiently explained terms like "PR" and "negative split," and turned me on to the miraculous healing powers of ice-baths and Ibuprofen.

People joke about how my running partners are a step away from an old folks home, but I know the only hope I have of catching these guys in a race is if I toss a cane or walker in their path to trip them as they fly by. Jack recently ran the Grandfather Mountain Marathon, touted as "one of America's toughest marathons." Forget beating them. I'm just trying to keep up.

As we run in the pre-dawn hours past darkened store fronts and traffic lights blinking yellow, we talk about everything from religion to politics, what was good on TV last night to how to fix the economy, and always, always, we talk about running.

My geezers take an active interest in my running career, for which I'm grateful. The first time I won my age group in a race, Dave, the ultramarathoner, saw the look on my face and proudly said "Oh, she's got a taste for it now." In my first marathon, I was running out of steam and despairing of making the time goal I'd set for myself when—as if from a dream at mile marker 23—Jack appeared. He suspected I might be flagging and fell in step beside me, encouraging me to push through the pain. With his help, I beat my goal time by 4 minutes.

At the end of our runs, Royce high-fives me, while Jack offers a more formal handshake to go with his quiet praise of, "Well done." Sometimes they say things like, "You had a good pace going," or "You looked strong." I'm as happy to receive these compliments as a first grader is having her drawing placed in the center of the chalkboard for all to admire.

A year of running has done the trick. My geezers tell me I'm improving. Soon, they say, the student will surpass the teachers. They seem pleased by this idea. I'm pleased as well. I have a competitive nature and, being truthful, I'd like their asses to be mine at mile 20.

But though I may someday whiz by my geezer comrades in a race, I realize after a year of training that there's more to our time spent together than just running readiness. Sure, I've learned how to work through a muscle cramp and how to drink water and keep moving. But they've also taught me lessons about patience and commitment, and what it feels like to accomplish something I once never thought possible. They've shown me by example what a difference it can make to have someone believe in you.

In one of those random conversations people have, someone asked me the other day what one item I would save if a fire were to break out in my home and I had only seconds to make a decision. I didn't hesitate in my response. I'd race to my exercise room and grab the plaque by my treadmill that commemorates the completion of my first marathon, and the celebration of friendship. Beneath the glass it reads, "Presented to Dena Harris, December 8, 2007. We Welcome You To The Marathon Club. Your Running Partners, Jack & Royce."

That first race is behind me and I have many more to come. But when it comes to matching the wisdom and friendship shared so openly and generously with me by these men, it's clear I still have miles to go before I'll ever measure up to their footsteps.

~Dena Harris

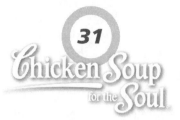

31

Give 'em the Knuckles

*It's a great feeling when someone like Bernard Hinault
comes up to you on the podium to say "Welcome to the club."*
~Lance Armstrong

Remember that scene from *Forrest Gump* when he's trying to find a seat on the bus and at each row someone says "seat's taken" or "you can't sit here." It's a pretty extreme example of how not to treat an outsider, but it is probably still pretty uncomfortable to watch for just about everyone, because we've all been there. Maybe we haven't been openly rejected like that, but certainly we've been in that spot where you're new to a club or a town or a group or something, and unless you're completely cold-blooded, you've always got at least a little desire to fit in somewhere, find where you belong. Sometimes we don't make the effort with the new guy because we don't have the time or energy to do the whole "welcome to the club, my name is so-and-so, did you find everything alright…." But it doesn't have to be that formal.

We learned that when we joined Juventus, our current bike club. We were new, nervous, excited about taking a chance at leaving the comfort of our old club. There were elite athletes around; people who knew real racing, how to dress, what to ride, how to win. We were just recreational riders and it was intimidating at first.

Now, right from the start we got a lot of help. We were fully welcomed by the established riders and coaches. I remember getting advice from one of the fastest racers around right before a big race, even though he had to prepare for his own race and take care of the rest of the team, and it meant a lot. Another coach invited us to train with the juniors when it fit our schedule better, even though he was busy getting the kids going. All of these gestures made a huge difference for us, but one really stuck out for us because it was at the very beginning, even though it was something pretty small.

At training in the winter, in the very beginning, there was always this one fast guy who trained with the elites. He knew everyone and was part of the main group. After each hard workout, he'd saunter over to his buddies and stick out his fist and they'd clank their knuckles on his, as if to say, "nice work." They "got the knuckles" is what we started calling it. Now, I don't need someone else's approval to feel good: I get what I want out of things, and we didn't view him as some sort of hero or anything, just a fast dude in the club, but we couldn't help wondering if we'd ever be part of the group like that.

Then one day, my wife came home from the workout. It had been a hard one and she was spent. She hadn't felt very strong and she might normally have been a bit down, but she was pumped. She was grinning from ear to ear. "So how'd it go?" I asked.

"I got the knuckles tonight," she said.

Then one night I got them. No grand gesture, no formal welcome, not even a word or anything. Just suddenly one night the fist was pointed at me. It made my week.

We joked about how "getting the knuckles" was some sort of secret handshake at the club and it was the only way to know you were in. We have a friend new to riding and she joined us at the club. Last week my wife came home and said, "Shauna's pretty excited; she got the knuckles tonight."

It really showed us how it doesn't take a lot of time or a big formal effort to make someone's day. So maybe next time you see someone new, maybe the new guy at work, or the new guy at your club, you don't have to take a lot of time to make them feel welcome.

Just go over and give 'em the knuckles.

~Tim Brewster

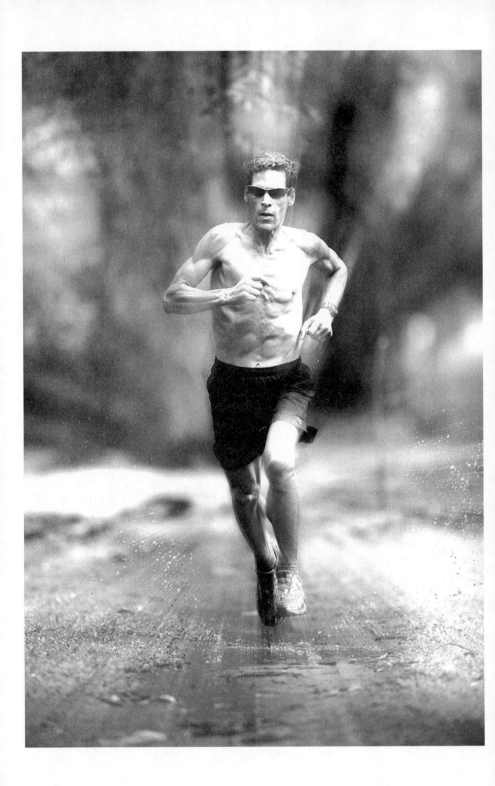

Runners

Comebacks

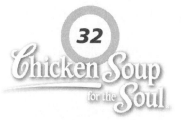

32

The New York Marathon after 9/11

We all stand together to help each other...
We remember forever all the brothers and sisters that we lost on that day.
~Rudolph W. Giuliani

T he New York Marathon is one of my favorites, but that year running it didn't feel so much like a choice as a necessity because two months earlier the Towers had been taken out. I got a call from a friend who was doing television coverage for the marathon. Because I currently held the world's best marathon time for female leg amputees, my friend thought of me for her segment, which would focus on non-New-Yorkers returning to the city after 9/11.

I agreed, because, like everyone else, I was looking for something helpful to do. I quickly sent out an e-mail requesting that friends donate dollars for miles. I got a thunderous Minnesota response and quickly collected thousands of dollars for the 9/11 relief fund.

I felt a bit sick as we flew in over the gaping hole in the New York skyline. Once on the ground I noticed something else that was different; people on the street were more open and vulnerable, making eye contact, initiating connection, showing they needed each other.

On Marathon morning, my friend interviewed me on the Staten Island side of the Verrazano Bridge, with almost 40,000 runners filling all available space, waiting for the ten o'clock start. It was a cool morning but people seemed to be shivering more from emotion than temperature. "In Memory Of" signs were pinned on thousands of runners' backs, and most of us instinctively huddled in groups. Plenty of runners get loose by mile 20, but never before had I seen so much crying before a race. Haze and grit hung in the air, but even though inhalers were tucked into jog-bra straps and waistbands, I think we were all aware of our good fortune to be alive and able to run through the New York streets.

There were groups of police officers and firefighters along the course. Both groups had suffered terrible losses, and we were all running in honor of them, with NYPD and NYFD hats and T-shirts peppering the crowd.

Being an amputee runner often invites attention and emotional connection—even with strangers. Prosthetic running legs look interesting, and their very existence represents resilience. This is the human way; we fall and with a little help, we get back up. Hopefully, we end up stronger than we were before. When people see my leg, they feel they understand something about me and seem encouraged to share something about themselves. As the race began, I fell in step with a young woman wearing a baby-blue T-shirt printed with a picture of a handsome young man.

"I'm running for my boyfriend. He was killed when the first tower came down." Her sentences fell to the ground, mixing with our steps.

"This would have been his first marathon. I thought I would be able to feel connected with him if I ran for him… it's so hard to be here without him, so hard to be anywhere, really…."

Her tears dropped and I couldn't speak, only able instead to put my hand on her arm.

"I know he would want me to do this for him, but I'm not a joyful runner anymore." Her last sentence toppled from her lips to join the others on the ground.

My pain for her and for all the others like her came out in a sob. She looked over at me and nodded, accepting what I had to offer. At some point we lost each other. I have thought of her often throughout the years, hoping she has found her way back to being a joyful runner.

I ran in and out of stories, the slapping sound of thousands of shoes on the road as background. Tears and laughter wove through the crowd. Applause broke out every time we passed a group of firefighters or cops.

Spectators were jammed in along the course. I knew when I crossed the invisible line between neighborhoods because Brooklyn accents switched to Jamaican, which then changed to Puerto Rican. As we crossed another street, Hasidic children with sleeves pulled down to cover their hands lined the curbs to give us high-fives.

My pace slowed as I ran into Harlem, where the gospel choirs stood on the stairs of their churches. A woman caught my eye, sent a big smile my way and in a beautiful Jamaican accent, called out: "You can do it, girl, you know you can!" Her friends joined in, and at that moment, I did know I could. On Marathon Sunday, it's easy to believe we can figure out how to live peacefully with each other.

I wasn't having a great leg day. At an aid station, I leaned on two firemen in order to get my prosthesis off, because there wasn't a chair or even an open curb to sit on. I finally broke the suction, pulled the leg off and smeared Vaseline on the raw spots. The taller of the two looked down at where the prosthesis had rubbed open a rather gruesome-looking sore, and groaned, "Oh, dear Lord. Does that always happen?"

I had to laugh because I knew this man had seen a lot worse, probably within the past week.

"Not always. I've had races where nothing opened up on me. Now, that's a good race."

His buddy chuckled at my tone and socked his friend in the arm.

"She's fine, Sal. Cut it out. She's almost good to go, aren't you, sweetheart?"

The firefighter, who wasn't much taller than me, but probably had seventy-five pounds more muscle, held onto my waist so I wouldn't fall over. Once I got my leg back on, he literally pushed me back out on the course.

"Make us proud. You're doin' what we all need to do."

I raised my hand, fingers splayed. They did the same. I ran on, feeling like I had made two new friends that, in all likelihood, I'd never see again.

I was still tightly surrounded by other runners as we made our way into Central Park. Normally I care enough about my time that I sprint the last quarter mile of the race, but this day, I almost slowed to a walk because my feelings overwhelmed me. I came across the finish line, sobbing. As I tried to catch my breath, I saw another runner doing the same thing. Our eyes met and we crossed the road toward each other.

"It's been so emotional, hasn't it?" I gulped out amidst my tears.

The tall, dark-skinned man wearing the NYFD cap made his own sobbing sound. We put our arms around each other and moved toward our race bags and warm clothes. We were only able to get out partial sentences, but they were enough.

"Did you see the fireman running with the picture of his station mates?"

"The one with his dog?"

"Oh, yeah, and did it feel to you like everyone wanted to talk?"

"Yes, and could you feel the energy when we went under the NYFD banners?"

"It was so sad and so hopeful all at the same time."

"And didn't you feel compelled to stop and hug people?"

"Yes, and I did."

We went silent then, wrapped in the glow of life, and the sadness of tragedy. We never exchanged names, we just cried together for the worst and for the best of humanity.

~Lindsay Nielsen

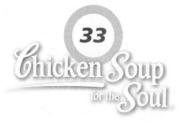

33

Triumph Over Tragedy

*The courage of life is often a less dramatic spectacle than the courage of a
final moment; but it is no less a magnificent mixture of triumph and tragedy.*
~John Fitzgerald Kennedy

Have you ever broken down a word and gotten results that
really defined the term at hand? I mean literally broken
down a word, phonetically and aesthetically and put the
pieces of the term back together and got something that is much
more simple to understand and easier to explain?

There are plenty of comedic examples of this practice but this
is not the venue for jokes. A serious example of this practice comes
from the word "triumph." Let's try it and see what we come up with:

First, we have "tri" or try, which means "attempt" or "have a
crack at" something. Next, we have "umph", when you say this with
emotion it signifies "hard work." In my life's experience, at times
as athletes (and non-athletes) we need that little extra "umph," that
push that tells us to "Cowboy Up" (any Red Sox fan circa 2004 will
get the reference) and sometimes competitors need family, friends or
the support of total strangers to push them a little further.

So let's break it down in a formal rhetoric:

Triumph—The positive outcome achieved when hard work is
implemented.

I first ran the Boston Marathon in 2002 during my freshman
year of college with my older brother Michael. It was a long race,
taking 4 hours and 15 minutes to finish; I was exhausted at the finish
line but not broken. I kept my shirt on for the first few miles and

eventually threw it on the side of the road in the ocean of other shirts taking advantage of the nice day for a marathon. On my chest was my name "SCOTT" in big bold magic marker written in my brother's handwriting for the verbal support of the thousands of spectators and total strangers from Hopkinton to Boston.

I saw my family and a few friends from high school and college along the 26.2-mile path and I got genuinely excited seeing a familiar face, but as the race went on and the adrenaline dissipated, faces got blurry and all I had to push me was self-determination, self-motivation and the screams of the anonymous spectators imploring me to "Keep on truckin', SCOTT!"

After finishing the marathon, I endured a few weeks of blisters and rashes. I had a good excuse to be late for my classes because I was moving so sluggishly due to tightened muscles and stiff joints. Overall, after the marathon recovery, I was as good as new; I was better than new! I felt such a sense of personal satisfaction that I decided for the rest of my tenure as a college student I'd run the Boston Marathon.

If the praise of friends and family wasn't enough, if knowing that I was the only student at my college who had even attempted (let alone finished) the marathon wasn't enough, if being able to walk my campus with my head held high and a glide in my stride wasn't enough... then mile 13 was enough! Mile 13, you may ask? Mile 13 was Wellesley College, an entire mile that had runners running by an all-women's college with a gorgeous female population cheering on the athletes pushing them beyond their pain.

That glorious day in 2002 was repeated in 2003 and 2004 and my plan was to complete the cycle and run it for a final time in 2005, but a careless, reckless and self-destructive decision I made in September of 2004 not only threatened to end my career as a distance runner but my life as well.

I was declared legally brain-dead on the night of September 18, 2004 because of a decision I made under the influence of alcohol. Miraculously I made it through that night. After three weeks in a coma, months in the hospital, years of physical therapy and intense physical conditioning with my good friend and personal trainer, Walter Laskey, I made it back. While I was in a coma my father made a promise by my bedside that if I woke up the two of us would run the marathon together, and if I were unable to run he would run for me.

Eventually, I was able to work my way out of a wheelchair and hobble around my house which soon evolved to hobbling around my yard which eventually progressed to going for walks around my neighborhood. In just two short years I was running—not particularly fast or with the best form, but I was running.

Soon after I started running, my father and I decided that we'd run the marathon, only not alone. My brother Jason who was a freshman in college, sister Jen who was a junior at the same school and her boyfriend Josh all decided that they'd run it too.

To most reasonable people, attempting a marathon would not be a feasible task unless they were given years to train for the race, but I already had three marathons under my belt and I've never been a reasonable man with a reasonable family. My family had pushed continually, every day and every night asking only for a full recovery. I am forever thankful.

The most agonizing part of my training was dealing with what is known in the medical community as "tone" (basically the constant locking up of a limb, in my case, my right arm). My tone, which only seemed to present itself during periods of exercise, caused me immense mental and physical pain. Eventually, after many frustrating runs and attempts to combat the tone by having my arm duct-taped or ace-bandaged to my chest to keep it from locking, I grew accustomed to the pain where it became more of an annoyance than a reason to stop running. I still battle tone today during periods of light to moderate cardiovascular exercise.

Only a few hundred yards into the race on April 16th, 2007 my arm locked up and stayed that way for most of the day. I can vividly remember "Team Maloney" (as we were called on the local news) arguing that we would stay together, but I knew that my younger brother, who was approaching his physical prime, would not be able to trot at such a slow pace for the duration it would take me;

same thing went for Jen and Josh. Not even my father, who was fifty-one, could go at my slow pace. My iPod was attached to my left bicep via an armband and my right arm was locked so I couldn't adjust the volume for most of the day. I had Aerosmith filtering out the sounds of the cheers, at least that's what I told myself. The truth of my story is that I was going at such a slow pace on such a cold, windy, and rainy Boston day that most of the fans were gone as I trotted by (I'm pretty sure a glacier passed me!). After the first few miles nobody could brave the elements long enough to see me. For me, 2002 was the year of the hare and 2007 was the year of the tortoise.

Everyone knows the story of the tortoise and the hare but the more realistic conclusion of the story should be "Slow and steady wins nothing… but will always finish."

My time nearly doubled what it was my first time out in 2002! When I was ambling ever so slowly by Wellesley College I was looking for a single spectator to verbally push me. But there was nobody there, either the weather was too fierce or I was just going too slow for anyone to think that there was still a single runner all that way behind the last herd of athletes… or a combination of the two.

As I crawled down Arlington Street and took a left onto Boylston (approaching the finish line), I could recall live bands playing shows for local radio stations in years past but not this year. This year as I went down Boylston Street marathon workers were already breaking down stages and taking down lights, but I had something waiting for me at the finish line, not a trophy or medal, something so much better, something that would last long after the medals are lost or hidden away in a drawer.

I had my family waiting for me at the finish line. That was all I needed, I knew that Jason, Jen, Josh and my father, mother, and little brother Kyle would be waiting.

My poor decision several years before had pushed me and my entire family into a marathon of a different kind, one they had not volunteered for or deserved. But that day, completing the

Boston Marathon marked the end of two marathons and a new beginning.

I had achieved success, I had prevailed… I had triumphed over tragedy.

~Scott Maloney

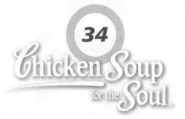

34

Racewalking

Your body is built for walking.
~Gary Yanker

After years of pounding my knees and ankles in dashes and the long jump, pain ended my decades of track and field competition. But how do you live without the adrenaline of racing? That's simple. You just become rational at age sixty and turn to competitive swimming! Suddenly, the pounding was gone, and so was the pain. And I was gone, too, in less than a month, bored by pool laps and no scenery. Now what?

A friend in the Annapolis Striders had the answer. This marathoner said he had stayed fit by vigorous walking while healing from a running injury. "Try it," he said, "It's even a competitive sport." Sure enough, a certain kind of energetic walking is a 100-year-old Olympic event called Racewalking. It's the most efficient way that a biped can move, and that shows in Olympic competition where winners of the men's 50K race will finish at an average of 7 minutes to the mile for those 31 miles.

I took to this sport immediately because there was no pounding involved, and thus no pain. Its special way of moving is so smooth that no cushioning is needed in the shoes. Many people use this method of striding just for health benefits. You don't have to enter races to be a racewalker.

However, those who compete must follow two rules and must please numerous hard-eyed judges or be disqualified (DQ). The first rule says one foot must be on the ground at all times. Horse racing offers a comparison: if a trotter breaks the required style in harness racing, and goes into a gallop, it gets DQ'd.

The second rule is designed to guarantee no running. How? Well, it's impossible to leap or jump or run unless the knee is bent to spring you up or ahead. Thus, on the advancing leg, a racewalker's knee must be straight at a given point in its movement.

Violation can cause a DQ. It took me many months to become fluid in the style.

But I was "off and running," so to speak. I took group-coached lessons from Dave McGovern, a world class racewalker. (To see his style in walking the mile in 6:00:72, visit www.racewalking.org and click any photo at the top of the page.) In time, I earned age-group gold medals in Senior Olympics' and USA Track & Field Masters' competitions. Hallelujah! I had lost a sport but had found another.

Then came a disaster. All the words in my saga start with "S." They surge, surely and swiftly, on a slippery slope. This sequence shows the segues: stride, stroll, saunter, shuffle, stagger, stop. The cause? Another "s": suffering. Lower back pain had arrived.

"Surgery is a last resort," I was told. But months of therapy didn't help.

The culprit was a slowly closing foramen, pinching a nerve passing through.

The cure was to enlarge that bone hole and relieve pressure. I saw it as akin to expanding the Holland Tunnel from the inside while traffic flowed. Some loss of leg control was predicted from nerve damage during removal of surrounding bone in tight quarters. I took the chance because the pain would only worsen.

Dr. Clifford Solomon, super-surgeon of Annapolis, Maryland, worked the cure. It left me with full leg control, but a flopping foot. I would be able to jog care free, but not meet racewalk rules. Months of therapy didn't help. My spirits sank to the level of that foot until by chance I tuned the TV to an old movie showing Fred Astaire dancing up a storm. From the ankle down, his feet swiveled like pivots, in the very motion I needed. I turned off the TV and went to the Senior Center.

As the only man among twenty-nine students in the tap dancing class I learned that grandmothers are programmed to care for any wounded creature. Some fussed over this seventy-five-year-old invalid, staying after class to guide and inspire. Many had been childhood dancers; some were from chorus lines. They were there to recapture lost skills. They knew the value of repetition on performance and muscle memory. And they knew how the magic of music can make therapy endurable and even playful. With example, humor, encouragement, advice and team drill-drill-drill, they taught me to tap dance. The guy whose wife always claimed he had two left feet had learned to dance. Those grande dames cured my flopping foot. I will be forever grateful.

Within a year, I was competing well enough to enter the USATF Nationals at Boston and break the American record for the 3000 meter racewalk. The article about my race is on the wall of Dr. Solomon's office, with a "thank you" inscription. And now, at eighty-six, I'm still competing and often thinking of dancing ladies.

~Charles Boyle

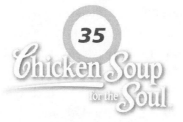

35

The Warrior Woman

That which does not kill us makes us stronger.
~Friedrich Nietzsche

My sister Mary is strong. She is not one of these girls who cries over broken nails. She doesn't cry. Yell, maybe, but not cry. A warrior woman whom I dared not wrestle, especially in front of my friends. She won awards for track and field as well as basketball in high school.

Then the accident happened.

Her boyfriend had been driving the car when the Ford F-150 swerved into their lane going over 70 miles per hour. It hit them head on, pushed them backward more than 50 yards before riding up over the top of her Toyota Camry, crushing the roof.

When I showed up in the hospital I didn't even try to count the tubes going into her. Her arms and legs were bandaged, as was her head. She was so thoroughly covered by bandages and blankets I could only see her face, which was swollen, but only from crying. She actually had been crying. That worried me more than the tubes.

We learned that the truck's driver and passenger had been drunk, and the passenger was killed when the truck flipped after crushing the roof of my sister's car. But Mary, strong as she was, survived somehow with only lacerated arms and legs, and severe nerve damage in her right leg and hip.

When the small car and the Ford F-150 smashed head-on, the impact was so great that Mary's seat belt burned through her dress, through her skin, and into the muscle and bone of her leg and hip. She learned that she'd need physical therapy even to walk, so bad off were her right leg and hip.

Ten years later, Mary was still picking windshield glass out of her forehead, arms and legs. She'd been dealing with the pain of damaged nerves in her leg, foot, and hip for a decade. Frustrated, she wanted to fight back against the pain, to assert herself that though wounded, she was a wounded warrior. And warriors don't pity themselves, don't dwell on what they can't change. Against her doctor's recommendation, she began to run again.

When my sister begins anything, she does not wade in. She dives in head first, clothes and all. In fact we've jumped off several high bridges that way. That is the way Mary went into running, the way she reclaimed herself, her strength, her soul.

Mary boarded a plane for Colorado in September of 2007. Her destination was the Colorado Marathon. After only training for it a few weeks, with a scarred, burning hip, leg and foot that seared with pain at every step, she ran 26.2 miles. And as soon as she crossed the finish line, she said, "That's it?"

Amazingly, the running helped. During the race, she'd been in pain for the first few miles, but her leg actually felt better afterward. Not having run many marathons, she was still finding her pacing, and after the Colorado Marathon she realized she still had plenty left in the tank. Her one regret, of course, was that she hadn't run harder.

My sister still runs, still has marathons on her mind. No one thought she'd ever be the same after that horrific crash. But in a sense we were right. She's not the Mary she used to be. She's even stronger. It took that crash for us to realize that it was never really Mary's body that made her strong in the first place. It was her unflinching vigor, her passion. If anything, that crash only made her stronger.

~Ron Kaiser, Jr.

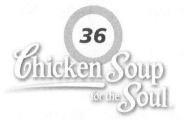

36

Bumps in the Road

Vitality shows in not only the ability to persist but the ability to start over.
~F. Scott Fitzgerald

I answered the phone, lost my job, and in one swift, silver-lining moment, realized my recent string of running injuries and lay-offs had been a gift.

When my boss called to say the company I'd worked at for twenty years was downsizing and my last check was in the mail, I discovered, as I stood there in the kitchen with the phone to my ear, that I was oddly and confidently prepared to handle this news and, in that instant, saw my running setbacks for what they really were — strengthening exercises. Lessons that could help me navigate the bumps in the road that is my life.

As I listened to my job evaporate, I got it. I suddenly knew what all the effort, discipline and disappointment had been about. "You've been an asset," said the telephone voice. As the platitude pile grew, so did my epiphany. Those injuries and training heartaches had made me stronger. They'd tested and toughened me, and they'd taught me how to take the long view.

I'd been running a long time. For years I'd go out and do my four miles, often feeling I could go on forever. One day I did, turning in a joy-filled, lactic acid-laden thirteen. I mentioned that outing to my son's basketball coach, an avid runner. "So, you did a half marathon," he said and, with that m-word, planted a 26-mile seed in my head. Before a week had passed, I was contemplating the possibility of going the whole distance and visualizing myself in a marathon T-shirt.

I signed up for a fall race and trained hard. Too hard. After a month of living by the training schedule hanging on the fridge, tendinitis got me.

I found out what a physical therapist does and made a mental note to always have one on my holiday card list. I learned the art and science of proper stretching, strengthening and buildup. My therapist healed me fast and got me back out there with seven weeks to go before the race. I'd cross-trained through rehab and had maintained a decent level of fitness. With work and a little luck, I could be ready.

On the first run of my resuscitated training program, I fell off a curb and suffered a third-degree ankle sprain that looked like a ripe eggplant. My family iced the elevated lump while I cried.

Before the end of this new layoff, I'd registered for a May marathon. With physical therapy, my ankle healed just in time to start training. A bitter winter set in, but I savored every crystalline run. I used an indoor track on icy days and spent one 20-miler running for three hours in a circle, direction changes the only relief.

Spring came. The long runs turned from frigid tests of will to sun-soaked communions with nature. I was mentally and physically ready. On my last truly long run, three weeks before the marathon, my left leg caved in. The physical pain was intense. The emotional pain of knowing it was over, again, was unbearable. I didn't need the official diagnosis of stress fracture to realize I wouldn't see the starting line.

When my daughter came home from school, she found me, leg propped on pillows, sobbing. Having seen variations on this theme, she knew what it meant and what it meant to me. She hugged me, took my hand, and said, "Don't worry. There are other marathons. You'll just try again, right Mommy?"

Perspective is a wonderful thing. My thwarted efforts to make it to a marathon had taught my daughter something about persistence, patience, focus. And faith. The busted leg didn't hurt so much anymore, and the wounded psyche felt a little hope massaging its sore spots.

I healed and started over. Six months later, I finished my first marathon. While finishing was euphoric, just being there was life-changing. Toeing that start line was a personal best that will never be trumped.

Fast forward to my kitchen. Phone in hand, I let my boss finish telling me how sorry he was about the job loss.

But I was already thinking about the future. I knew I'd land on my feet and toe the start line of some new challenge. As there are other marathons, there are other jobs.

The world brims with possibility. Once you're confident about your potential, there's no race you can't run.

~Lori Hein

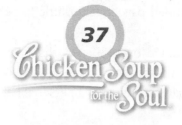

37

A Runner

I run because it's so symbolic of life. You have to drive yourself to overcome the obstacles. You might feel that you can't. But then you find your inner strength, and realize you're capable of so much more than you thought.
~Arthur Blank

Anyone who has taken up running for the fun of it knows nothing compares to the high you get when you've pushed through "The Wall" on rubbery legs, miraculously feeling nothing but good. For me, each step I took even when I didn't feel like it provided a sense of inner strength and wellbeing. Running allowed the physical world to slip from my consciousness, my mind astoundingly untangled personal problems, even unraveled the puzzle of world peace from time to time.

Since the age of six I'd competed in sports. Competition filled my life with small achievements that felt big. I started running in college after a lifetime of grueling swimming practices came to an end. At first, running was my antidote to fries and beer. However, it didn't take long to get hooked—especially when my running route wound through unique urban neighborhoods that surrounded the University of Pittsburgh.

One neighborhood was characterized by the mansions of long-gone steel magnates. The next was defined by rundown row houses young people were rehabbing. A canopy of trees covered the sidewalks and provided just enough shade to keep me going through the second pass of my five-mile route. It didn't matter that at least three months of every year were marked by frigid temperatures. I was that much stronger when spring finally sprung.

My running wasn't confined to where I was living at any given time. Each vacation or visit with friends became a running discovery zone. Sunny St. Helena in the northern California wine country, Laguna Beach, Carmel, Lake Tahoe, Philadelphia, suburban Maryland, Tucson, and Kiawah Island. Each place proudly shared its hidden treasures. When I think of running in those places, different feelings are instantly evoked—specific to the place. As though I'm there.

Running made me feel part of the place I was visiting—instantly a community member. It also created and nurtured relationships. My husband and I ran races together. Friends and professors in my Ph.D. program found running bolstered opportunities to learn as though our minds worked better when our bodies were in motion.

Shortly after my thirty-fourth birthday, running came to a screeching halt. Admitted to the hospital with debilitating numbness, pain, weakness, and fatigue, I was diagnosed with Multiple Sclerosis (MS). As much as I wanted to go for a run when I left the hospital, I couldn't.

My leaden body disappointed me repeatedly. It took all of my energy to care for a baby and a toddler. That feeling when you have the flu—you can't get off the couch and if you do, you're back on it in 20 minutes wondering what you thought you were trying to prove—plagued me. Even with help from family members, breaking out of the cycle of fatigue and pain to start running again wasn't happening. Nothing was the same.

Mentally, this was disastrous. I was a runner. An exerciser. Not a couch potato. Suddenly, exercise was my enemy. Instead of runner's high, I had runner's remorse. Wouldn't life be easier if I never felt my mind unwind while moving through space at the speed of light? Okay, I never ran very fast, but I could go long. I needed that back.

More than two years have passed since my rapid spiral into what felt like my ninth decade of life. The MS symptoms have lessened. Much of my life is back to normal. I've been walking and trying to run. One foot in front of the other. Should be so easy. But searing pain in my feet, as though a vice is closing on my bones, forces me to stop after only a few steps. I stumble. Sometimes literally. Mostly I trip over the fear I'll never be my old self. Am I damaging my body if it's so hard to run?

The scientific answer is no. It's better to be in shape when the next episode comes along and dares me to live my life the way I want to. I still think of myself as a runner. Even though I'm not. Walking doesn't provide the Zen-like state I'm chasing like water in the desert. I wish it did.

I'm not giving up. I can push through this. "The Wall" every runner knows so well may be a little thicker for me, but the exhilaration will be that much greater when I finally manage to recapture Running. Boy, will that be good.

~Kathleen Shoop

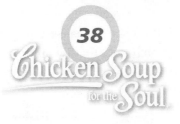

38

Why I Run

*I have always thought the actions of men
the best interpreters of their thoughts.*
~John Locke

llow me to introduce myself. I am a long distance runner who logs 140 to 200 miles per month. People are very passionate about running: they either love it or loathe it. I run seven days a week.

When I was fourteen, as a cyclist, I was hit by a car and almost paralyzed from the waist down. I spent the next four years wearing a back brace complete with custom steel rods.

I began running seven days a week to strengthen my core muscles. It was grueling but my persistence paid off. I built my core muscles solid and was able to shed my back brace before I graduated from high school.

When I was twenty-five, I was in a car accident in which I herniated the disks above and below my now degenerating vertebrae—another setback. Being stubborn and determined, however, I ignored the doctors who told me to limit my activity and again set out to rebuild and strengthen my broken body through my own personalized training program. That impairment only cost me two years.

When I was thirty-one, I was in yet another car accident in which I tore both of my Anterior Crucial Ligaments—another hindrance. That injury was serious. I had surgery and underwent physical therapy three to five times a week due to complications. It took me two years to learn how to walk again, having to wear knee braces every day during that time. The specialists told me that their goal was to get me to walk "normally" but that I would never run again—devastating news for someone who views running as the oxygen she breathes.

The doctors were right. For the next nine and a half years, I was unable to run more than twenty-five feet without my knees ballooning up like cantaloupes. Having four children by then, it was extremely frustrating to not be able to rise to the athletic ability I was used to.

In 2006, I began self-training to participate in a 60-mile, three-day breast cancer walk. My goal was to accomplish that task blister-free, without inflamed knees and feeling strong at the end. I began a self-guided five-month training regimen. I was determined to do that event without the use of my knee braces. Yes, I still needed to use them while engaging in sports. I knew I would have to build my core muscles strong to support my back, as well as my leg muscles to support my knees.

Three months into preparing, I realized that walking four to five hours a day was too time-consuming. If only I could jog part of it—that would abbreviate my time spent training. I started jogging between telephone poles without my knees swelling. Slowly and cautiously, I increased the distance. Two months later, I was up to running six miles without my knees protesting. Being highly competitive, I relished proving the doctors wrong. Of course, it only took nine and a half years to do so.

While practicing, I suffered a devastating loss, a dear friend—my senior by one year—suddenly and inexplicably died. His life's mission had been to mentor women to accept themselves and reach their fullest potential. He firmly believed that people should let nothing hold them back from attaining their goals.

Soon after his death, while on one of my runs, a crazy thought entered my mind: what if I could run the LA Marathon? I remembered viewing that event on television as a child, thinking that the people who crossed the finish line were gods. I wanted to be one of those gods. I wanted to know what it felt like to traverse the prized finish line, even if it meant I had to crawl across it.

The seed was planted. I had only four months to get ready. I took my self-taught training to an all-time high and prepared as if my very existence depended on it—actually, it did. I knew that if I didn't train to my fullest, I would tear my body apart and the doctors' diagnosis would win. I wasn't about to let that happen. I was on a mission: I would run the LA Marathon to honor my fallen friend and fulfill one of my life's greatest goals. I trained eight times a week, seven days a week—twice on Wednesdays. I dedicated my final quarter-mile sprint of every run to my lost friend, as a way to remember his teachings and life's work.

My hard effort paid off. I celebrated my friend's memory by sprinting across the finish line of the LA Marathon strong and solid—he would have been so proud. Since then, I have crossed the finish lines of many marathons, half marathons, 5Ks, 8Ks, 10Ks, 12Ks, obstacle courses and Mud Runs all over the United States to the amazement of my doctors. I select one individual for whom I run each race. This is my way of honoring the tremendous physical or emotional impediments they are facing, or for those who have lost their battle and passed on.

I'm often asked why I run, to which I always reply, "I run because I can, for those who no longer can." Through my own personal mantra, "Just take it… embrace it! That's why you're here," I remind myself that the aches and pains I experience while training and racing are nothing compared to the suffering those whom I revere must endure. This is why I run.

~Cindy Hanna

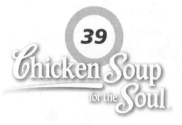

39

Dreams

Follow your dreams, for as you dream you shall become.
~Author Unknown

Everyone dreams.

Mary Peck's dream was to make it to the 2004 Olympics in Athens. She was a great runner, and certainly had every right to believe she could make it.

At the tender age of twenty, her confidence was only surpassed by her talent, and Mary had this uncanny way of making all who knew her believe too.

Mary also suffered from an eating disorder. She was anorexic. Unnaturally thin. Mary lived with the continued emotional pressure that goes along with this condition. It consumed her. Through it all, Mary ran. Running became her oxygen, her reason for living. And marching with the athletes at the 2004 Summer Olympics was her goal, ever-present in her mind. She trained every day as though she'd already made the team. If you called her and got her voicemail, you'd hear, "Sorry I'm not here to receive your call personally, but I'm out training for the 2004 Olympics. Wish me luck and leave a message."

I became Mary's chiropractor in early 2001. In addition to her eating disorder, she also had a chronic back problem. I often wondered if her back pain was a by-product of her emotional pain. Either way, Mary responded well to having another person care for her. She'd come in three times a week for treatment and our standard five-mile run, while her grandmother who drove her would sit in my waiting room and wait for us to return. I needed the training, making this the perfect co-dependent relationship.

Some days were easier than others. On a good day, we'd chat and laugh, just like old friends would do. On not-so-good days, we'd be silent for six miles. I often wondered what she was thinking, as the silence would sometimes be distracting. But, I practiced silence on these runs, and usually let Mary dictate how much conversation we'd have.

There were two hiatuses in our relationship. One in 2001 and another in the spring of 2002. On both occasions, Mary went to Arizona to an eating disorder camp. Both were expensive, but those who loved her were excited she was going. After the first camp, Mary seemed better. Upon her return, she smiled and talked more on our runs. Unfortunately, this change would slowly fade.

In early 2002, Mary returned to Arizona for a second tour of the camp. Our hopes were that more was better, and each visit might add to her prior gains. Upon Mary's return from her second visit, she was great. We all held our breaths with optimism.

Until that bright and sunny June day when Mary and I had a treatment and run scheduled. "Mary, what would you like, four or five miles?" I asked. "You decide," she stated. For unknown reasons, I chose five miles. But, this particular day, I cut our five miles short as my wife, Trudy, wanted me to run with her when I returned to the office. I asked Mary if she minded cutting it short, and of course, she didn't. That was Mary. Surprisingly, this was the first run in many months that Mary responded positively when asked how she felt. I smiled. We finished our run, said our goodbyes, and Mary left with her grandmother.

The next morning, while at my computer working, Trudy gasped at the morning newspaper. There was a picture of Mary's bicycle helmet and two state troopers. "20-Year-Old Cyclist Killed By Dump Truck." My mind raced; what time did I run with her? Could it be another Mary Peck? Regardless of the questions, none of the answers helped. When all the dust settled, the truth was evident; this was our Mary.

Mary's grandmother had let her out of her car halfway home to ride her bike the rest of the way. Tragically, Mary was hit by the right front end of a dump truck. She was killed almost instantly.

From an Olympic hopeful to a fatality in the blink of an eye. Needless to say, I couldn't help but wonder, what if we'd run the full five miles? Or, what if I had decided four miles from the start?

Mary had made many friends in the running community in her short lifetime. The trials she faced and the fight within her every day made all of us proud beyond words to have been a part of her life. Why this could happen to someone who fought so hard, there were just no answers.

Mary's family elected cremation with final residence in the wall at the National Cemetery. The following Tuesday, one week after my final run with Mary, I re-ran the same course. This run re-defined the word "alone."

Dreams are bigger than life. They can make the impossible become possible. Most would have cried and accepted Mary's tragic ending as her final chapter. Not her dad. "I watched Mary prepare every day of her life for the opportunity to march with the athletes in the opening ceremonies of the 2004 Summer Olympics in Athens, Greece, and I wasn't about to let it not happen," said Richard Peck.

Richard Peck is a pilot. Surprisingly, he had an opportunity to fly another female Olympic swimmer to a destination that she "had" to be to. She was so worried she wouldn't get there in time, and it shocked her that someone would willingly fly her there on their own time. She could never have imagined the resolve in the heart of Richard Peck to help Olympic athletes. "How can I ever repay you?" was all Richard needed to hear in order to implement his plan for Mary.

The plan was that the captain of the soccer team would be the one to represent Mary. Mary was also a star soccer player in high school, and this was the perfect arrangement. This plan fell apart when the soccer team wasn't able to take part in the opening ceremonies due to a game scheduled at the same time. This "problem" opened the door to a much bigger opportunity.

Dawn Staley, a three-time Olympic Gold Medalist, a member of the WNBA All-Decade Team and the current head coach of South Carolina was selected for the greatest opportunity imaginable. She would be the flag bearer for the United States in the opening ceremonies. She would lead our country into and around the stadium.

On August 13, 2004, Dawn Staley and Mary Peck met for the first time. They led the country in the marching of athletes at the opening ceremonies of the 2004 Summer Olympics in Athens, Greece. Richard Peck provided Dawn with a heart-shaped necklace holding a small container with Mary's ashes, as Dawn proudly participated in the greatest event on Earth. Everyone who knew and loved Mary cried and smiled while watching such a spectacle.

No one could have written this story, or even predicted this turn of events. However, Mary Peck made it to the marching of the athletes at the 2004 Summer Olympics, just as she had dreamed, proving once again, dreams do come true.

~Dr. Tim Maggs

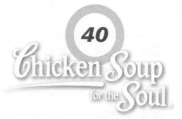

40

Through Grit Alone

The difference between the impossible and the possible
lies in a man's determination.
~Tommy Lasorda

T he only thing going through my mind was "hang on." I didn't have any brilliant near-death thoughts or see any flashes of light. I had been riding on the back of a pickup truck with my buddies from the summer landscaping crew when the impatient driver of an 18-wheeler tried to pass us. He didn't make it past us in time to avoid the narrow bridge ahead. When he tried to get back into his lane, he struck us, and I went flying over the side of the truck.

There wasn't even time for one of my buddies to grab me. I tried my best to keep my grip on the side of the truck, but my fingers slipped and I tumbled down to the pavement. Attached to our pickup was a trailer that held three tons of lawnmowers. My leg got stuck in a brace on that trailer, which meant that I got dragged down the hot Georgia asphalt for 324 feet before the truck came to a stop.

When at last all was quiet and still, I could not move. My leg was trapped in the brace, with all the weight of that trailer resting on top of it. The trailer was acting as a tourniquet: if anyone moved it, I would bleed to death.

My best friend, looking ghostly pale, came to attend to me while others went to phone the hospital and my parents. I was just eighteen years old, and this was the summer after I graduated from high school. Instead of having the time of my life at college with my buddies, I was going to spend most of the next year on an operating table or in a hospital bed.

Drifting in and out of consciousness for those first couple of days meant that I had no real handle on what was happening to me. I knew I'd been in an accident and I knew it was pretty bad, but it did not occur to me that there might be any permanent damage. I was shocked, then, to hear a doctor's voice in the background saying to my parents, "We're going to have to amputate his legs." My parents negotiated with the doctor to save one.

Surgeons removed my right leg. Unfortunately, the left leg would never heal correctly, not even after two dozen surgeries. My heel bone had been ripped off, and no matter what they tried to do to reconstruct one, it was never quite right.

For years, a traumatic brain injury left me lost and drowning in depression. I lost count of how many prescription drugs I was taking, chased by alcohol. My glory years as a high school athlete were long gone. Now I could barely run around a track without my left foot opening up and getting infected, landing me back in the hospital. I couldn't stand for any length of time.

It took twelve years before I made the decision that would get my life back on track: I had the other leg amputated.

In no time at all, I found that I had an uncanny ability to balance on my new prosthetics, and that I was able to do much more now with no legs than I was with my one "real" leg. But I felt like I was living what Thoreau called a life of "quiet desperation." There was no vision, no purpose. I made God a deal: "Open a door for me and I will run through it!"

Weeks later, I browsed through magazines in a bookstore and saw two stories that gave me the answer to my prayer. One was the story of Sarah Reinertsen, a single-amputee who had just completed an Ironman triathlon race; and the other was the story of a soldier returning from Iraq missing one of his legs.

Though the circumstances were different, the young soldier's story was similar to my own. I wanted to do something to help others like me. I had never heard of an Ironman triathlon, but as I read Sarah's story, something lit up inside me.

It's known as the toughest one-day endurance race in the world; a 2.4 mile ocean swim, then a 112 mile bike ride through the lava fields, then you warm up for a marathon: a 26.2 mile run. Each discipline is timed and you must complete it in seventeen hours. I had no business even thinking about it — I didn't know how to swim, had never ridden a bike with prosthetics, and since my accident I had never run even .2 of the 26.2 miles that I would have to run. That day changed my life; I finally had a direction. I was going to do this crazy, unthinkable thing.

The best successes are achieved with lots of support, and I was lucky enough to have a whole team of people get behind me. Not only did I have no legs, but I was also overweight, bordering on diabetes, nearly forty years old, and broke. All I had going for me was sheer grit. My parents thought I was crazy, but a local swim coach offered to help train me after-hours in a high school pool, and a local spin studio owner taught me how to ride a bike. My prosthetist worked on customized legs for me after hours and for free. A fellow triathlete offered to become my manager and help raise sponsorship money to get me to Hawaii for the Ironman, and others offered to train with me.

Shortly before the race, I broke a vertebra in my back during a bike accident, and a bad person stole my running legs. Training was brutal, but despite it all, I felt such a sense of hope.

October 13, 2007 was the big day. With a good-luck kiss on the cheek from my on-site coach, I waded into the water… and got kicked in the eye almost immediately. Now not only did I have no legs, but I was also blind in one eye. Still, I got through the swim. The winds were so strong that I was almost knocked off my bike several times, and I was disoriented and weaving by the time we got to the run, but after dumping pools of sweat out of my prosthetic legs every few miles, I crossed the finish line with only 17 minutes to spare.

"Scott Rigsby, you are an Ironman!" the announcer, Mike Reilly, called out. "The first double-amputee in the world to finish the Hawaiian Ironman."

It would take weeks for my body to heal from all the injuries it sustained, but the memory of making history and changing the world would last a lifetime. Unthinkable? Yeah, right!

~Scott Rigsby with Jenna Glatzer

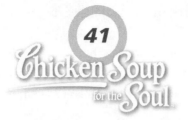

41

Deena Kastor

*If your actions inspire others to dream more, learn more, do more
and become more, you are a leader.*
~John Quincy Adams

Deena Kastor is one of the greatest women distance runners in the world. In addition to winning the bronze medal in the marathon at the 2004 Summer Olympics, she is the American record holder in the marathon (2 hours, 19 minutes and 36 seconds) as well as in the 10,000 meters (30:50.32).

However, it is more than fast times that in my eyes make Deena a true champion and role model. Let me share with you Deena's trip to the 2007 Track & Field World Championships in Osaka, Japan, where she competed in the 10,000 meters.

Deena went to the World Championships with the realistic goal of standing on the medal platform. However, she didn't have her best race by any measure and finished a disappointing—for her—sixth. So instead of a medal, Dena received heartbreak. And yet when she was interviewed right after the race, when her disappointment was at its max, Deena made no excuses and graciously congratulated the other runners. This again was not amazing though, because Deena is always gracious in victory and defeat.

No, here is the amazing thing Deena did. Two days after her disappointing race in Osaka, she returned to the United States with her husband, Andrew, but instead of feeling sorry for herself for a bummer of a race, Deena was already thinking about others who don't even have running shoes much less races to run in. Specifically, she was thinking about the underprivileged (in truth, NO-privileged) children from inner-city Los Angeles, to the Dominican Republic, to Sudan, Uganda, Liberia, and Kenya, to whom my "Share Our Soles" (S.O.S.) organization sends used running shoes so they can enjoy this great sport that helps provide confidence, self-esteem, friendships, and strong character—you know, so kids can be a little like Deena.

Before they even arrived at their Southern California vacation beach house in Oxnard, Deena called me to say she had another batch of running shoes for S.O.S. for me to clean up and then send off to underprivileged youth in faraway lands. The truth is, the shoes Deena donates don't require much cleaning. They are almost like new; some, in fact, are brand new.

I created S.O.S. five years ago after a hip stress fracture and then serious knee problems sidelined me from running track and cross country my freshman and sophomore years in high school. Though heartbroken, I knew I would eventually get healthy and run and race again, but I started thinking about kids who can't enjoy the great sport of running not because of injury but simply because they don't have running shoes. To date we have collected and donated more than 4,100 pairs of running shoes to needy kids. Deena and Andrew have been my biggest supporters, donating more than 300 pairs by themselves.

Deena does more than just unlace her shoes after a few weeks and a couple hundred miles and toss them in a bag. She also collects them from many of the world-class runners she trains with. Andrew, who is a personal trainer, collects shoes from his clients. And then they pack these smelly shoes in their car and drive them all the way from Mammoth Lakes to Oxnard for me to pick up. Of course they offer to deliver them to my door, but I always insist on coming to get the latest haul, which is always a thrill because they invite me in for a long visit.

Obviously, I want to talk to Deena, who is nicer than words can describe, about her amazing career. But she and Andrew, who is equally friendly and warm, would rather ask me about my training and racing—for Ventura High School during the first two years after I met her and now for the cross country and track teams at the University of Southern California where I'm a sophomore. In truth, we end up talking a lot about everything but running.

During my pick-up visit just a couple of days after her 2007 World Championship disappointment, Deena apologized because she said she left some near-new running shoes in her hotel in Japan. On purpose. She explained that the housekeeping staff would be able to take the shoes—as well as some clothes and backpacks she left behind—home to their families. To me, that is Deena—a champion not only on the track, but more importantly a champion in the sport of life.

Indeed, being a champion does not necessarily mean winning a gold medal or even a bronze. As greatly as I admired Deena after she earned a bronze medal in the 2004 Olympics, my admiration grew further still after her heartbreaking—rather, bone-breaking—race in the 2008 Olympic marathon where she was forced to drop out after less than five miles because of a stress fracture in her foot. Typically, Deena did not react with anger or self-pity. She met with the media and was a portrait of grace and dignity. Rather than dwell on her own misfortune, Deena looked beyond her own setback to help others; shortly upon returning to United States she gave me another load of running shoes for S.O.S. As I said, Deena proves one can be a champion without breaking the tape, without standing on the medal platform, even without crossing the finish line.

I have a framed autographed picture of Deena hanging on my wall with the inscription: "Greg—Keep inspiring! Continue making a positive difference in all you do!"

Truly, those words best exemplify what Deena Kastor does—and not just after a medal-winning race.

~Greg Woodburn

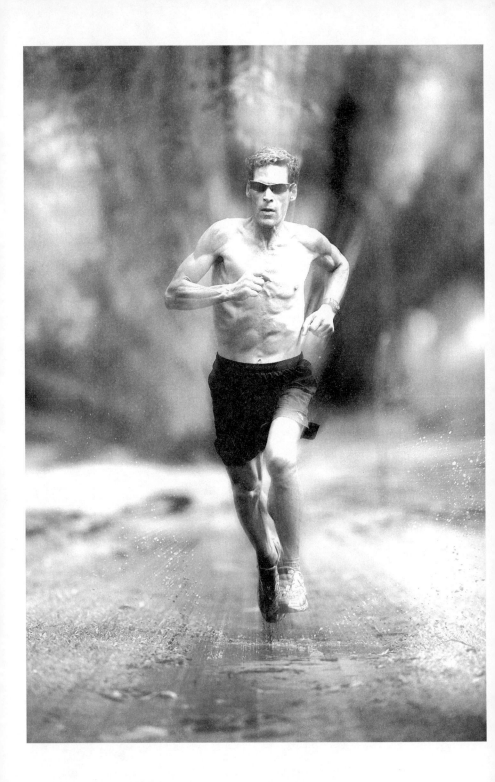

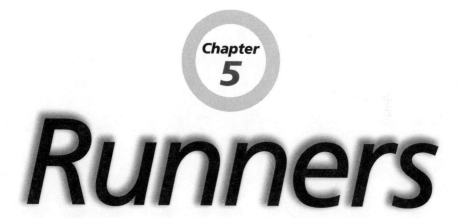

Chapter 5

Runners

Everyday Adventures

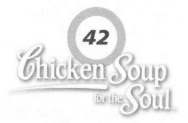

42

Miracle on the Run

Miracles are a retelling in small letters of the very same story which is writ-
ten across the whole world in letters too large for some of us to see.
~C.S. Lewis

W e experience miracles every day, thing is, we're just too busy to see them. But every now and then a miracle is so big and bold that it's unforgettable. Truth is, most days aren't mountaintop experiences, most days I find myself longing for miracles; days when I'm down and discouraged, crushed and cast off, days when I want to overcome but just feel overwhelmed—on days like that I remember days like this.

It was early summer, 2004. I was training in Murrieta, California—a town about 60 miles northeast of downtown San Diego. This training cycle was sandwiched between my 7th place finish at the Olympic Marathon Trials and my US Team appearance at the World Half Marathon Championships in India.

As a professional runner, my training regimen calls for both morning and evening runs. Once every 10 days the schedule calls for a glycogen depletion run. In laymen's terms: I run until my accessible energy stores are totally zapped. This means a 25-30 miler at no faster than six-minute mile pace. Long run days are great because there's no second run. One and done.

On this day, I woke, drank my coffee, read the paper and prepped for the run. Just before noon I walked my coffee out of the comfort of my 69-degree house onto my porch to check the conditions. When you live 20 miles inland in Southern California you never know when the warm winds from the Santa Ana Mountains will blow through. When they do, it feels like God left His hairdryer on. This day He left it on high.

I considered postponing the run until the late afternoon but not being one to let a perfectly good caffeine buzz go to waste, I figured I would brave the high noon elements. Most days I drive the course and stash bottles every three or four miles but out on my porch I had a thought—no, an epiphany—I could do this long run without any fluid support.

I realize most humans would never consider, much less attempt, running over 20 miles without fluids but as a professional athlete I am, at times, delusional and lose touch with my mortality. Now, through therapy, I can admit that I have a bit of a superhero complex. I mean, I can string together a series of sub 4:40 miles, I've run 50-mile races, I've run 25 miles with no fluids before—I could do it again. I can leap tall buildings; I can run through walls—you see how this superhero thing can prove problematic.

So I set out in my shorts, shoes and MP3 player, and despite the heat, I was in the zone. As every runner will tell you, every so often the stars align and everything comes together. On those days you can do no wrong, you can do anything, you feel like a superhero. I passed the mile in 5:19—way too fast.

I hit five miles just under 27 minutes—three minutes too fast. So I did what any reasonable athlete would—I changed my music from the long run mellow mix to techno-Rocky and let her rip. I started hammering, faster, faster, faster.

On long run days I like to run out and back courses. This way I can't cut it short. One way out and one way back. At the time, this route was pretty desolate. It traveled along Winchester Road and headed out toward a town called Hemet. I don't know much about Hemet other than it smells like cows and it serves as a shortcut to Palm Springs.

I was hammering along the dirt shoulder and passed 10 miles under 53 minutes—right around five-minute pace for the last five. I reached 12.5—the 25 mile turn around—but things were going so well I figured I'd run the full 15 and try and set a personal best for 30. I reached 15 in under 1:23 — six-minute pace for the last five. I was slowing, but still feeling good.

The next five passed without incident but the naked sun in the naked sky was relentless; the rays pounded my shoulders. I began feeling the effects of the heat. I reverted back to the slow mix and slowed the pace in an attempt to preserve the effort.

That's when things started going wrong, real wrong. Anyone who has run in the heat will tell you, things can go from good, to bad, to worse, to you're totally screwed in about the time it took you to read that sentence. Pardon the juxtapositional phrase but *things tend to snowball in the heat.*

I was still managing seven-minute miles but was slowing by the second; this was becoming a death march. My mouth was dry, my throat was dry, I tried to swallow — nothing. I couldn't spit; I was no longer sweating; pasty white sweat covered my chest and arms — I was dehydrated.

I wasn't a superhero — I was an idiot. Only a fool would try and run 30 miles in horrible heat with no water.

Reality: I am susceptible to the same natural laws as everyone else. People need water. Runners need even more.

I kept running, using the term loosely now, and began licking my arm. And before you laugh or cringe, don't knock it 'til you try it.

The wheels were coming off, there wasn't anything around, and to top it all off, in all my years of training I'd never failed to reach my destination. My running rule, and life rule for that matter, is "keep moving forward."

So, I started to pray. Nothing pious mind you, I was just talking. "Lord, I'm really stupid. I'm in a lot of trouble here. I still have a long way to go and if I don't get some water I won't make it home. So if you could hook me up I'd appreciate it...." I paused, then added, "Maybe you can have someone pull over for some directions and give me water."

I run around 50 times a month, which over the course of the

year makes for roughly 600 times I lace up the shoes and pound the pavement. Out of those 600 runs a passerby will stop to ask me for directions five times, maybe six on a leap year. People assume runners know the area, and truth is if you are looking for a street and it's the runner's home turf, they're essentially a walking, talking MapQuest. So I figured offering the direction suggestion was a solid scheme to give the creator of the universe.

I continued running and for the next minute continued offering up all sorts of ways He could deliver me some fluids. "Someone could get a flat, one of my friends could drive by, a fan could stop for an autograph, a girl could stop for my number." They were all solid suggestions and things that had happened in the past so I figured I'd give God a hand, you know, in case He was short on ideas.

A minute later a blue midsize pulled off onto the dirt. My water had arrived.

The car stopped about 30 feet in front of me. I stopped the music and slowed to a stop. A lady exited the car and approached.

When I stopped I felt a cold rush to my head and felt like I was looking through a zooming camera lens—in and out, in and out. I lost my balance and fell forward. Fortunately, my hands preserved my pride and I saved myself from falling. Of course, being an egomaniac too proud to admit he had fallen over, I played it off like I was doing a hamstring stretch. I stayed bent for a few seconds and waited until my equilibrium returned. The woman's feet appeared in front of me; I rose out of my jackknife.

"Are you OK?" she asked.

"Yeah, just stretching."

I should have said no and begged her for a ride but superheroes don't need rides.

"Do you know how to get to Pechanga?"

Pechanga is an Indian reservation—a gambler's paradise—think Vegas in Cali.

"What you need to do is head back that way, get on the 15 South, it's the second exit, you'll see the signs from there."

"Thanks!" She started walking away. Apparently God forgot to tell her she was supposed to offer me water.

"Um, Miss? Do you have anything to drink?"

"Lemme check."

She walked to her car, returned with a bottle. "I took a sip," she said, "is that okay?"

I smiled, nodded, and graciously accepted.

She drove away. I walked to a tiny dirt cross street and took a seat on a small patch of dried grass next to a wire fence. I'd rest up, enjoy the water and rally for the last seven miles.

I thanked God for the hook-up and finished the bottle. I sat baking in the sun, trying to convince myself that once the water had a few minutes to absorb I'd feel better.

A minute went by, then two. I was fooling myself; I needed more water. So I prayed out loud, "Lord, thanks for the water but I'm going to need more, if you could have another car stop and give me a…"

As the words left my mouth a car turned onto the dirt road beside me. Chills ran over my body. I couldn't believe my eyes. Oh great, I was hallucinating.

I wasn't delusional; the car was real. I was so happy I could have cried, and probably would have if my body had any fluid left.

I stood, approached the car and the window rolled down, "Would you like some water?" the man asked.

Holy Shnikeys. I stared in disbelief. Crazy. Incredible. A miracle.

"Yes."

He got out of his car, popped the trunk and the only thing inside was a lone six-pack of bottled water.

He handed me one; I drank it.

"Would you like another? I have six."

"No, this will be fine."

He smiled.

"Sir? Why did you stop?"

"My son has a soccer game on Diaz Road and I can't find it."

"I think Diaz is on the other side of the freeway."

"Thanks. Have a good run."

I should have asked him for the whole six-pack but I was dumb-founded. I sat, drank, stored the two bottles next to the fence, went on my way and although I didn't break any records that day, I made it home.

Temperatures had topped 100. I stepped on the scale. I had lost 17 pounds—things nearly went very, very wrong.

That night I drove back down Winchester; my headlights caught the small green street sign next to the fence where I had sat—Keller Road. I grabbed the bottles as a reminder of my miracle on the run.

~Josh Cox

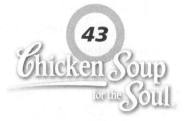

Nowhere to Go

Running is an unnatural act, except from enemies and to the bathroom.
~Author Unknown

It was a beautiful Sunday afternoon in early September. The marathon was only a month away and I was in the midst of a grueling training regimen. On this particular day I was scheduled for a fourteen-mile run, the longest I would have all week. So before I left, as always, I did some light stretching, ate a small snack, and of course, drank plenty of fluids. Soon enough I had my sneakers tied, headphones covering my ears, and was out the door.

The conditions were ideal for running—temperature in the mid-60s, clear blue skies, and a gentle breeze. With autumn knocking on summer's door I wondered if there would be many more days with such wonderful weather. I headed west towards the city center, seven miles one way, seven miles back. I reached the downtown high-rises with my body relaxed, my lungs breathing in a perfect rhythm and my legs feeling as strong as ever. But then, suddenly, out of nowhere, just as I reached the halfway point, I had to go.

It comes as no surprise, when running for hours at a time, that one would have to relieve oneself at some point. Normally it's not much of a problem, especially if you were lucky enough to be born a male, as I was. You simply jog off to the side of the road, find a concealed area, usually some bushes, and proceed to conduct your business. But on this day it was different. I was in the middle of one of the largest cities on the West Coast. There were no bushes or shrubs, only open sidewalks and exposed brick buildings. And on top of that there were people everywhere, strolling the city streets, enjoying the sunny day. I'd run myself into quite the predicament.

I headed back towards my apartment and with every step the feeling in my body became more intense. I began eyeballing side streets and alleyways, but with little luck. There always seemed to be a person walking around, or a slow-moving car in the near vicinity. Damn this beautiful day, I told myself. If it would only start raining, that would clear the streets and give me some privacy. But the sun continued to shine and the people laughed and smiled, as if they somehow knew what I was going through and were in on the joke.

I came upon a fast food restaurant and knew that they would have a bathroom inside. On the men's room door there was a sign that read, "Restroom Key at Front Counter." I patiently waited in the short line. When the people in front of me were finally done ordering I very nicely asked the cashier for the bathroom key. "The bathroom is for customers only," she said. "If you want to use it, then you will have to purchase something."

I tried my best to explain my situation. "I'm out training for the upcoming marathon," I pleaded. "I don't have any money on me, but if you give me a break, I promise to come back later and buy something."

"Sorry, paying customers only."

I wanted nothing more than to scream, but was afraid that it might make it worse. What was the world coming to? Is there nowhere to go to the bathroom? I continued east. My muscles felt fine, but the faster I ran, the worse it got, so I had little choice but to keep a moderate pace. Everything around me seemed to be a reminder of the situation I was in. There was a woman watering her flowers with a garden hose. And a man washing his pickup truck. Then I saw a dog lift his leg on a fire hydrant and almost lost it. It was probably the only moment in my entire life when I actually wished that I were an animal.

Finally I felt like I couldn't hold it any longer. I saw some bushes in front of a house and considered taking my chances. But then I looked around, and if it wasn't just my luck, there was a police department directly across the street. I weighed my options. On the one hand I really had to go, but on the other, how would I ever explain being arrested for such a foolish thing?

In the end I decided to hightail it home. I was only a couple of miles away, and ran faster than I had ever run before. I probably set a personal record that day in the two-mile, and when I finally arrived at my apartment I could have been the happiest man on Earth. I frantically searched my pocket for the door key and then fumbled around trying to insert it into the slot. I slammed the door behind me and sprinted through the living room. At last I reached the bathroom, and of course, it was locked. My roommate was taking a shower.

~J.M. Penfold

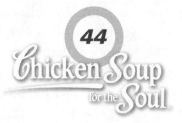

44

How Not to Jog

If you can look at a dog and not feel vicarious excitement and affection,
you must be a cat.
~Author Unknown

"So you're going for a run?" This from my husband the skinny engineer and non-runner.

"Yes. I thought I'd take the dogs."

"All three of them? Is that wise?"

"I don't know if it's wise or not, but that's the plan." This from me, the elementary school teacher who's trying not to slip into the disappearing waist, puffy thighs, flabby abs, end-of-youthful-figure zone, and who only started running recently.

I grab the leashes. The kind made of slim cords that extend with a flick of a button from a thin plastic handle. The dogs start slobbering. Jumping. Vibrating. Whining. They won't sit still while I put on their collars.

"Can you help me?" I ask my husband. He's watching me with an amused grin on his face.

I should explain here about the dogs: two Labs, Nate and Duke; one Border Collie, Jessie. They aren't exactly sterling choices for a peaceful afternoon jog. Two have never been to obedience school. One flunked out. And I rarely even take them on walks.

But we are all collared and leashed and ready to go. I've even done my pre-jog stretches. "I'm going to get a good workout today," I tell my husband. "I can feel it. Lots of cardio-building, thigh-busting exercise."

He smiles again.

"Okay, open the gate." I hold onto the leashes with a death grip, two handles in one hand, and one in the other. The three dogs hop and yip and foam at the mouth.

"Are you sure?" my husband asks.

"Yes, I'm ready."

He slides back the latch and begins to open the gate.

Larry, Curly, and Moe nose through and take off like rockets, dragging me behind them.

The wind rushes past my ears, and I hear the faint sound of laughter behind me.

Okay. This is not the plan. "Whoa!" I yank back hard. All three dogs jerk to a stop. Jessie, the meekest of the three, sits down and looks slightly guilty. "Walk!" I say, forgetting that this is supposed to be a quiet afternoon jog.

"Have fun," my husband hollers after me.

"We will!" I wave and smile. And the dogs jerk me onward.

We half-walk, half-trot down our long driveway. Then we turn left, onto a winding blacktop road, and settle into a brisk jog, the boys in front setting the pace.

My normal route is down this road, which runs past hayfields and then into an area with pristine woodland on either side, and back again. A nice two-mile jog full of the clean-air smells of the country. Unless you come across roadkill. That roadkill being a mashed-up skunk.

Now there's something about dead animals that I realize is terribly interesting to dogs. Especially mine. Before I can say, "Don't even think about it!" all three dogs are wallowing in the remains of the dead skunk.

I scream. I jerk. I stomp. I scream some more. The dogs run circles around me, tangling me in the thin nylon cords of their leashes, always going back to the skunk.

A pickup truck headed our direction stops beside me as I'm untangling myself. "Need any help?" the elderly driver asks.

I shake my head. "No thanks. I think I've got it under control."

The dogs wag their tails when they hear the man's voice. They whine and try to jump on his truck, like the man is their long-lost owner, and I'm just a ranting stranger. "Cut it out!" I yell. The man drives away.

I reel in their leashes as short as possible, and we finally leave the dead skunk behind, but not the smell. It lingers in the fall air and makes me gag as the dogs jog in front of me.

We're almost to the end of the road, where the woods are thickest and where I plan to turn around and head back, when I hear a noise in the bushes beside me. A loud, crashing noise.

The dogs hear it, too.

They stop. Ears prick high. No more panting. They all three stand like statues, staring in the direction of the noise.

And then it's there. A deer. A large deer. A large running deer.

My dogs take off. Straight for the woods. I pull back on their leashes and scream, "No!" I dig my heels into the soft leafy soil.

They keep going. "Stop!" I holler. Whatever made me think I could take three large, powerful, slightly overweight dogs on a collective jog? I must have been crazy.

I'm skimming across the ground now, leaning back, digging ruts with my feet, and they're still pulling me. Through weeds and briars.

I sit down for leverage. They keep running. Now I'm bouncing along on my bottom. I feel dirt sliding up under my shorts. My backside starts to burn. I bump across the ground, screaming. But I don't dare let go of the leashes.

"It's gone," I yell. "The deer is gone!" But the dogs don't believe me.

Finally, my feet hit a fallen limb, and we stop. The dogs are shaking all over. So am I. My heart is pounding, I'm drenched in sweat, and I think I have enough dirt in my shorts to plant a small garden.

I stand, rearrange the leashes, and take a quick look around. Then, as discreetly as possible, I yank down my shorts and dump out the dirt. I find a few biting fire ants mixed in with the dirt. And I think I have stickers in my butt.

I pull up my shorts. "So much for a nice peaceful jog," I say to the dogs. "Thanks a lot. I hope you're happy." They wag their tails at me like they are extremely happy.

I limp home with the dogs. They strain against their shortened leashes, and my arms feel like they're being yanked from their sockets. When we get to the dead skunk, though, I'm ready. We walk far around.

At home, I turn the dogs loose in the backyard. I will bathe them in tomato juice later.

I drag myself inside.

"How was your jog?" my husband asks, looking over his newspaper. "Dogs do okay?"

"My jog?"

He nods.

"I wouldn't be lying if I said it was interesting."

"Yeah? Get your heart rate up?"

"Yep. Did that."

"Feel like you got a good workout?"

"Oh yeah." I rub my hand across my backside and feel the prick of splinters. "Except…"

My husband sniffs in my direction. "What's that smell?"

"Meet me in the bathroom with a pair of tweezers. I'll explain everything then."

~Sharon Van Zandt

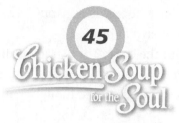

45

Morning Run

I love the sweet smell of dawn —
our unique daily opportunity to smell time,
to smell opportunity —
each morning being, a new beginning.
~Emme Woodhull-Bäche

I awaken with thoughts
of things to do today
I try to shut them out
but sleep will not return
I look out through the blinds
The morning star is visible
In the dark sky turning pink
I stretch on several layers
of comfortable clothing
Pull on my favorite old sneakers
Take from a drawer my MP3
Open the front door
Step out into the cold air
and stretch
I start immediately
Up a hill
And feel the exhilaration of adrenaline
Pumping through my body
Towards the top of the hill
My calves begin to burn

But no matter
The pumping music
Keeps me going
Around the block
And to the second hill
Now I feel like I can
Keep going forever
The week ahead of me
Beckons with hope
It feels great to be alive
Then around the last bend
Where I start to slow down
Just in time,
I think,
My body can't take much more
And home again
To the smell of
Freshly brewed coffee.

~Elizabeth Kathryn Gerold-Miller

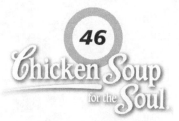

The God of the iPod

There is something powerful in Metallica, a will, a drive.
~James Hetfield, Metallica lead vocals, guitarist

I don't like to complain, but I'm going to anyway.

This winter has been pretty crappy. I can handle running in the cold, but ice is something else. The stuff is treacherous, especially for a guy with a couple of bulging discs in his lower back that don't respond well to wipeouts. Needless to say, I was thrilled when it finally started to melt.

It took until the second week of April before spring finally made an appearance in Calgary, Alberta, and it was a most welcome event because not only did it clear away the ice, it opened up my favourite running route that I had not accessed since the previous November. Because of the buildup of snow and ice, the run up Shaganappi Trail to Nose Hill Park had been impassable, so I had altered my course to travelling around my local neighbourhood. Admittedly, it is a nice neighbourhood, but nothing beats Nose Hill for the view, trails, and wide-open spaces, so I was understandably excited to be lacing up my runners one Good Friday.

The temperature was around ten degrees Celsius, but there was a brisk wind as I headed out the door, which made me wish I'd worn a thin hat—not to keep my ears warm, but to keep my stupid iPod headphones from being ripped out of my ears. I've heard other people make this same complaint about the headphones that come with iPods, and either our ear holes are too big or they make their ear buds too small. I crammed them in tighter to the point where it felt like they were pushing on my brain and ran towards the intersection of Country Hills Boulevard and Shaganappi Trail.

There had been much road construction in this area and the median had yet to be covered with sod, so I pranced from dry dirt patch to dry dirt patch avoiding the mud bogs as much as possible. Mud is the only thing I hate more than ice for running; at least ice doesn't stick to your shoes. I was almost through the minefield when I blew my right foot off, metaphorically speaking. I missed a step and sank into a pit of goo that crazy-glued its contents to the sole of my shoe. I hate that.

I looked down in disgust and missed the light to cross the eight lanes of traffic, so I took advantage of the several minutes it takes for it to turn green again by scraping the gunk off my shoe against the curb. Then I dragged my foot through some leftover snow much like a dog with worms will drag his butt across the carpet. It took the entire time that the light was red to get my shoe clean enough so that I wouldn't be unbalanced and running like a drunken Quasimodo.

I handled that little setback, so it was time to resume running up the monster hill I affectionately refer to as "The Bugger." It's two kilometers long and heavy with traffic, but it's the only way for me to get to Nose Hill, so it's worth it. Also, the nice people who built the road when it was twinned the previous year gave me an eight-foot-wide shoulder to keep me a safe distance from the motoring public.

The shoulder was covered in gravel that was a necessary evil to keep people from sliding sideways down the hill during the winter, and within half a kilometre a small rock had found its way into my shoe, so I stopped to remove it. Two hundred metres later another rock got in my shoe and I removed that one too. A few hundred metres more and there was a third rock and I just said to hell with it and let it stay.

Then a car sped through a large puddle that splashed me right in the face. I've run in pounding rain before, so this wasn't exactly a big deal, but what annoyed me was that it coated my sunglasses with mud and I was wearing one of those silver-impregnated anti-stink shirts that wouldn't exactly work for cleaning the lenses, so I would have to settle for an obscured view of the Rocky Mountains when I reached the park.

Finally I made it to the park and the wind was so brutal that, no matter how much I crammed, my left headphone would not stay put. What's more, although it was a sunny day overhead, the western horizon was obscured, meaning no view of the Rockies. Oh well, there was still a nice view of the city.

The trails were still too muddy, so I stuck to the paved bike path but soon had to detour around a newly formed lake of melted snow. Unfortunately, I stepped onto some grass that was more like swampland and let's just say that all the remaining mud got washed off my right shoe.

I sloshed and squished the next kilometre and then spotted a group of people standing and chatting. They were too involved in their conversation to notice their Rottweiler leave them to charge toward me, upper and lower teeth bared, a menacing growl escaping its throat.

My first reaction was to blurt out a blasphemous phrase that wasn't at all appropriate on Good Friday. Then I yelled at the owners, "Call him off!"

I don't want to get into the conversation that resulted, but the dog was very reluctant to return to its owner, and the guy acted like I had just spat in his soup by being concerned over his dog biting me. The woman with him, who professed to be a "radio personality dog trainer," said I was giving off too much energy and the dog was reacting to that. Uh, hello? Out for a run here. Expending energy is the whole point. If I stopped and calmly waited for every dog that crossed my path to come and sniff my various places, then my runs would take a lot longer. Besides, the owner obviously missed the sign that said the pathway is an on-leash area. The whole exchange left me aggravated and I started thinking about carrying pepper spray so I could blast some irresponsible owner in the face the next time his dog came at me.

I left them behind and futilely tried to keep my left headphone in place. When I reached my turnaround point I opted to tackle a muddy trail rather than risk facing Cujo and his brain-dead owner again, and while on said trail a cute chocolate Lab puppy charged toward me, tongue, tail, and entire body wagging. Obviously he posed no threat, or so I thought, until the forty-pound bundle of joy leapt off the ground, turned sideways in midair, and slammed his torso right into my chest, almost knocking the wind out of me. The woman who owned him chuckled and said, "Oops, sorry. He's just a puppy."

No kidding.

I was almost out of the park when a puffy, partially domesticated rat creature on about forty feet more leash than was warranted got it in its head that my ankles were the enemy. I was so miffed at this point that I just leapt over top of the sorry excuse for a canine and kept running.

I started running down The Bugger towards home and was rewarded with having survived thus far with a decreasing of wind that allowed me to listen to music in stereo for a change. After the frustration of the run I wanted to just let gravity take over and fly down the hill at a high rate of speed. I always found this good for an adrenaline rush, but with all the gravel I worried about a wipeout that would turn me into a giant, throbbing scab, so I kept my pace moderate.

As I neared the traffic light I judged the timing and saw that there wasn't much hope of making it through and opted to slow my pace and wait it out. I was annoyed with the entire outing and just didn't feel like going for it.

Then fate intervened.

I'm not sure if there is a specific god that controls the randomness factor of an iPod Shuffle. (Has Steve Jobs achieved deity status yet? I may have missed the memo.) Anyway, "He" decided that the next song that came up at that precise moment in time was one that would not allow me to choose anything other than going for it.

"Gimme fuel. Gimme fire. Gimme that which I desire."

Metallica exploded into my head, and without even thinking

about it my legs started pumping at full throttle. I was going to make that stupid light or get creamed by a car in the process.

It was a hundred metres away, and I sprinted like a teenage boy whose girlfriend's parents came home unexpectedly. The light turned yellow before I reached the first curb, but I pressed on across the eight lanes with a heartbeat that would be considered at maximum were I twenty years younger. I made it to the other side just as it turned red and celebrated my triumph by leaping over a construction barricade rather than choosing to go around it.

And I landed in a hole and my ankle turned on its side.

Did I mention that I broke both my ankles when I was a teenager? No? Well, now you're informed.

Then something amazing happened: My ankle snapped back into place as my momentum carried me forward. I barely paused as I realized that no damage had been done. I kept sprinting toward home, Metallica egging me on.

"Quench my thirst, with gas-oh-leeeen-UH!"

I ran across the field that took me to my cul-de-sac, leapt a fence, made a clean landing, and sprinted down the road and up the stairs of my house, bursting through the front door, dripping with sweat, heart pounding, lungs burning, and Metallica still blaring.

I read my wife's lips as she said, "How was the run?"

I smiled and between ragged breaths said to her, "Awesome."

~James S. Fell

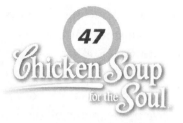

47

Waterworks

Laughter through tears is my favorite emotion.
~Steel Magnolias

I slowly made my way to the finish line. The baby rolled in my large belly and I had to stop until she finished adjusting.

"Only four weeks left," I reminded myself when she finally settled in and I started off again. "Come on, or we'll miss your dad," I told my three boys. We were going to support my husband as he ran his first 5K.

We found a spot where we could watch the runners cross the finish line. My boys ran circles around me as we waited. I felt like a sun with all my little worlds circling around me. No wonder pregnant women feel like the center of the universe, I was large enough to have my own gravitational pull.

A ripple went through the crowd as the first runners came into view. I looked at the time clock and my jaw dropped. I couldn't believe that someone could run so fast. I watched as people cheered for their spouses and children and kids cheered for their parents. There was this surge of emotion and everything in view started swimming as my eyes filled with tears. I was so proud of each runner.

"You made it," I'd yell and clap as they ran past me.

One lady was struggling. "You're almost there!" I encouraged.

Then my husband came into view. "Cheer for Dad," I told my boys.

They lined up and started yelling, "Go Dad! Yeah Dad!" their little hands clapping hard and fast. If I had been holding back the tears before, I couldn't now. Watching my boys cheering for their hero struck a chord and, while my smile was as wide as the race was long, tears streamed down my cheeks.

Craig crossed the finish line and found us. I kissed him in congratulations and he wiped my cheeks. We both laughed off the tears as hormones. I may have been emotional, but after three other pregnancies I'd learned to laugh at myself.

"Next year I'm running with you," I told him.

So the next year we lined up together with the other runners. This time I had butterflies in my tummy and no matter what I did they wouldn't settle down. I had been running for a couple of months and felt ready to run 3.2 miles, but the whole race atmosphere was new.

The course wound through a small town—past the church and school and through a couple of neighborhoods. There was only one hill to climb and that was at the start of the last mile. I could do this.

The race official yelled, "On your mark," and my adrenaline spiked.

I heard her yell "Go," and it was all I could do not to break into a sprint. Craig took off and stayed thirty feet ahead of me for the remainder of the race. I wasn't really worried about beating him—because there was no way it was going to happen. I focused on regulating my breathing.

I'd been going steady for about two and a half miles when a little boy and his dad came running out of their house and started cheering for the woman ten feet ahead of me.

"Go Mom!" the boy shouted as he pumped his fists in the air. Mom smiled and waved with both hands. It was so touching that my heart opened up and tears fell out. I was crying—again. Arg! What was with me and crying at races? I slowed down as my breath came a little harder. I hit a button on my iPod and a hard pounding song blasted into my ears. I shook myself—literally—and was able to keep going.

I hit the hill and climbed it like a champ. I was feeling so high. I headed around the last turn and had the finish line in sight. Right next to the timekeeper was Craig and he was yelling for me. I was so happy and proud that I started tearing up. I reached down and found the reserve I'd held and sprinted to the finish. I ran past him and took another twenty feet to slow down. I stopped for just a moment and leaned over to catch my breath.

"How was it?" Craig asked as he rubbed my back.

I looked up, showing the tears on my cheeks, and saw the concern on his face. "What's the matter?" he asked.

"Oh this?" I wiped the tears from my face. "I always cry at a run." He shook his head and laughed at me as I laughed at myself.

I've run many races since that day and there hasn't been one that I haven't cried at. I never know when the tears are going to strike or what will set them off. Kids cheering for their parents do it to me every time. Other times it's feelings of gratitude for what my body is able to do. Sometimes it's just the feeling of accomplishment as I beat my last time. They are good tears—tears of pride, of happiness, of hope, of admiration—I guess I get emotional when I run. I'm not usually an emotional person, but running gives me such a high that I can't hold back.

So I'll see you at the races—I'll be the one with a box of tissues.

~Christina Dymock

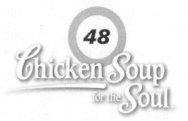

48

Keith's World

There is no time to think about how much I hurt; there is only time to run.
~Ben Logsdon

My brother runs. Not for office. Not for a cab. Not because he is late for an appointment, but for fun. He took up marathon running in his early thirties. He claims that a co-worker needed a training partner and so he tagged along as a favor. I didn't think too much of it until he casually mentioned during a Sunday afternoon phone call that he had entered a half marathon. After that Keith was hooked. One race turned into another and it wasn't long before he signed on for the entire 26-mile deal, the 2007 Columbus Marathon.

While admiring Keith's commitment to the sport, I admit that I know little about it, and lately I've begun to question his sanity. How do you explain a man who is almost completely devoid of body hair? He shaves his head completely bald on a regular basis. I assume it's for some aerodynamic purpose like a bicycle rider's helmet, but what about the waxed shoulders? Keith's shoulders are unusually smooth. He wouldn't confirm it but his wife did. I'd bet money his legs are next. I never knew you could gain on the competition with less hair. Painful? Probably. Time consuming? Definitely. But my brother runs for fun.

Water intake is incredibly important on race day. Too little water and the body cramps. Too much water and it sloshes around in the stomach, possibly causing nausea. Keith miscalculated his hydration needs during the 2009 Chicago Marathon. He drank too much water; not enough to make him sick, but enough that he had to detour every few miles off the course for a pit stop. Kind of like a race car I guess. I wish I had been there to see the look on his wife's face as she cheered him on only to watch him run for the bathroom, disappear for 30 seconds, then jump back onto the course as though nothing had happened. As I've learned through numerous conversations with him, water intake is a fluctuating science in the runner's world. My brother runs for fun.

According to Keith, there exists a love-hate relationship with carbohydrate ratios which is partly scientific and partly Las Vegas luck. He burns about 3,000 calories on race days—thinking about it makes me want to faint. Keith must carefully choose the kinds of carbs he'll consume and accurately calculate a consumption of 500 to 700 grams per day on training and race days. Can someone convert that to ounces? Even more confusing is the idea that not all carbs are created equal. Simple carbs and complex carbs are very different. Only those that the body can convert to glycogen are useful to runners. Does that mean chocolate is out? I could never live without my chocolate. I've heard that sports gels, or energy gels as they are commonly called, are quite helpful if your stomach can tolerate them. Keith's stomach prefers to yak them back out, as I think mine would do if I were eating souped-up energy and nothing else. He is still experimenting to discover the best balance for his body. Fortunately, he only runs for fun.

Speaking of queasy stomachs, Keith admitted that many runners routinely yet involuntarily lose the contents of their stomach. He himself has thrown up in more than half of his races. In one particular half marathon, Keith threw up four miles into the race. With nine miles to go he pressed on determined to finish. Runners he had passed near the beginning were now passing him as he struggled with his stomach. A mile from the finish line he finally caught up to a group of three and passed them for the last time. With a quarter mile to go and another competitor bearing down, he felt his stomach turn. He dug in for a final burst of energy, stayed ahead of the other runner, crossed the finish line and promptly threw up in front of several hundred people. I can't decide if his strategy was dedication or pure insanity, but from my perspective it was certainly gutsy. Good thing he just runs for fun.

Aside from the science of hydration and carbohydrates, I'm really blown away by the amount of training that goes into preparing for marathons. Keith once told me that he runs 300 to 400 miles to prepare for each race. I honestly don't think I've run 300 miles in my entire life. That's a lot of miles. Then there's the constant speed battle to improve one's own personal time. My brother runs a 9-minute mile for true marathons and a 7.5-minute mile for half marathons. That seems fast to me. As I recall, the last time I ran a mile for any reason was when I thought a bear was sharing the trail with me at Glacier National Park. It was 1992. I ran straight down the mountain to the parking lot and into the safety of a friend's car. I had been hiking for fun but the bear changed my mind.

I'm puzzled by mounting evidence of Keith's love affair with the medical community. There's the orthopedic doctor with whom he's on a first-name basis, and his physical therapist who he too addresses by first name. He spends $400 on custom-made orthotics for his Asics which are also made by an orthotics specialist. For that kind of money he had better be on a first-name basis. He schedules regular visits with his doctors and specialists more often than I book spa appointments. After running 26 miles, maybe he books a spa appointment too. For a man who waxes to streamline airflow, it's entirely possible. Keith did say recently that he sweats so much while running that the salt crystals on his face dry into a fine white powder, which I can only imagine must provide additional seasoning for his carbohydrate-rich sports gel. Hmmm. I wonder if that too is part of the fun.

Although I did not grow up in a runner's world, I have grown to appreciate all he has endured to develop into a competitive weekend athlete. I may not always understand the science behind the sport or his enjoyment in running for hours at a time, but I love the Sunday afternoon stories he shares that bring us together across the miles. Thank goodness Keith runs for fun.

~Jenny R. George

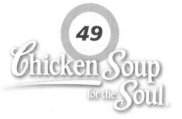

49

The Truth about the Winter Runner

Running is a four weather sport.
~Author Unknown

In Siberia they call it the "breath of stars." It happens when temperatures fall so low in winter that condensation from the breath solidifies into ice crystals before it hits the ground. Here in Minnesota it isn't quite that bad, but there are times—during a particularly long winter's cold snap—that it does feel like we are clinging to an existence north of the Arctic Circle. Of course, this is a point of pride for most of us. We scoff at those who set off for warmer climes when the going gets tough. Folks who trundle off to exotic places like Miami or South Padre Island where less-fortified Midwesterners can wear their flip-flops in December and not feel ashamed. These people are Minnesotans according to the Census Bureau only. If they come back for a Christmas visit sporting tan lines and bleached hair we know they're not really one of us no matter where they pay their water bill.

If we're really truthful, however, even those of us warped enough to stay in the frozen north all year long would much rather snuggle up with an electric blanket and a hot toddy than venture out into a frozen February morning unless we absolutely have to. After all, there are limits, even for us northerners. The only people who are the exception to this universally-held sign of common sense are those who feel the need to get up in the dark, cold morning, risking life and frostbite to go for the dreaded early-morning jog.

Frankly, most of us who are not runners simply don't get the concept of running for joy in any kind of weather, let alone when it's cold enough to solidify anti-freeze. On a very personal level, I'm not sure I could be convinced to run even if I was escaping a burning movie theater. Therefore the concept of a daybreak dash or a January jog is anathema to me and my brethren. Yet there are people—and plenty of them—who are up at dawn, running on ice and snow with an abandon few of us mortals can comprehend. We see them as we commute in our cozy SUVs, leaving an ever-bigger carbon footprint on Mother Earth without allowing our shoes to actually touch the ground. Oh yes, we snicker, we sneer, we honk from time-to-time. We point and giggle and laugh at their folly. And when we arrive at work, we gather together at coffee breaks to hoot about the "health nuts" we saw flinging up snow in their wake a few hours earlier. Yet somewhere lurking deep in our psyches there's something more, something we're often afraid to confront and would probably admit only under the most hideous torture. Somewhere deep within our condescension lies a smattering of admiration.

Yes, admiration. Like a couch potato sports fan, many of us secretly look up to those who do things we know we could never do, or for that matter, would even attempt. Much like hang gliding off Mount Everest, most of us would never dream of awaking, pre-dawn, bundling up in a jogging suit, duck down vest and knitted cap to run for fun in the snow and slop. Ice is something for gin and tonics in our secure little world, not something to be tread upon before the *Today Show* hits the airwaves. Yet despite our barbs and finger-pointing, those diehards who get up and run mile after mile before heading off to work or school do have a measure of our respect whether we wish to admit it or not. Consider this, then, a tip of the hat to those who don two or three of them for their daily morning run. You may not convince me to join you on your morning jog, but I'm beginning to look at your tireless efforts in a new, not-so-condescending way, even if I can't bring myself to admit it during my 10:35 coffee break.

So keep up that pre-dawn, winter jogging routine. And forgive the rest of us for our snide comments and stinging remarks. Understand that, deep down, you have our admiration for the kind of tenacity you have that the rest of us just don't seem to possess. It'd be nice, too, if you could keep in mind that we're not really snickering when you tell us there's no such thing as bad weather, just bad clothing. It's an act we must put up to fit in with the non-running crowd. Underneath it all, we know you're right.

~Mark Spangler

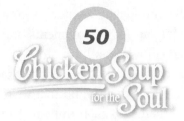

50

Cleansing the Soul

Everyone who has run knows that its most important value is in removing tension and allowing a release from whatever other cares the day may bring.
~Jimmy Carter

The crisp air stings my face. While I lace my shoe, she circles me with anticipation. The sun winks a sleepy greeting and I stretch my arms to the clouds above me. I breathe in the fragrant morning and exhale with intent. It's time to begin. I move forward and she responds, taking the first steps in this well-practiced routine that never ends the way it begins. My footfalls are heavy next to hers. We struggle to find rhythm in this dance we've done a hundred times. Our warm breath escapes in front of us.

The smell of licorice tickles my nose while dawn creeps up on the still and silent Earth. The hillside glistens with dew; the skyline, freshly painted, meets the mountain's outline. The colors are more vibrant than at any other time of the day. I'm breathing deeply, and I slow our pace. She is always too anxious in the beginning. I hear my shoes on the pavement and the clinking of her collar.

It isn't long before we find our stride and move in unison. I feel my body lighten as the worry and stress of life falls from my shoulders and is carried away by the breeze. My faithful partner runs silently beside me, often glancing in my direction. Is she happy? Is this process as healing for her as it is for me?

Now moving as one, I loosen my hold on her leash. I relax and extend my limbs. Momentum carries us up and down the country hills effortlessly. I feel like I am floating and my mind is flooded with thoughts and ideas. I notice the sounds of birds now echoing in the trees. The sun has fully risen and beams down. Deer stand statuesque in the distance, watching us. I'm thankful for their quiet stance; she doesn't notice them.

We follow our well-worn path and sometimes find a place of euphoria, unexplainable and intoxicating. Our pace quickens and the air no longer feels cold against my skin. We are lost in time. Time is not always my own, but in this moment, it is. Only I will say how far I go and how long I run. There are no interruptions. No demands on my time. When I run, I am not Mrs. or Mom. I am a writer, a runner. Limits only exist if I've set them for myself. She is content just being with me.

This moment carries me deeper into a sense of self. I feel I could run forever. However, life awaits my presence. We slow our pace and begin our journey back. Now, free of all burdens, I am inspired by the day; I am ready to take on all that life might throw in my direction. Slowing to a walk, I take a deep breath and release her. She hesitates to leave my side.

I whisper "go home." She, so obedient, turns and runs up the drive.

As I take my final steps through this ritual, I reflect. I feel strong and energized. Renewed. Running, my addiction, has worked its cleansing magic on my soul once again. I am now ready to enjoy what I love most—being a wife and mother.

~Machille Legoullon

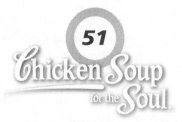

51

Initially I Was Alone

I feel the earth and the wind and the trees.
I feel its spirit. It puts me in the moment.
~Gabriel Harmony Jennings

I arrived at the scheduled time of 7:30 AM
The entrance to the parking lot was closed
I would have to wait on the street for my training partners
The fresh blanket of snow might have prevented them
    from being on time
I would wait 10 minutes before beginning my run

Shortly after starting my run, I realized I was not alone

Maybe it was the crisp morning air kissing me on the cheek
Maybe it was the beautiful snowflakes passing my eyes
Perhaps it was the bird chirping in the winter woods
Or was it the sound from the peaceful trickle of the stream?

Maybe it was the gentle sound of the new snow under my feet
Maybe it was the sound of the snow as it fell from a giant
    oak tree in the frozen forest
Perhaps it was the brilliant path illuminated by the snow
Or was it the cascading of the waterfall over the Glen?

A wide grin came across my face
This was a day the Lord had made

I rejoiced and I was glad
Initially I was alone, but I very quickly realized
My training partner is always by my side

~Gil D. Hannon

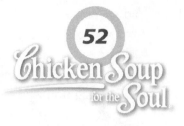

Race Day

Everyone in life is looking for a certain rush. Racing is where I get mine.
~John Trautmann

I began channeling Constantina Dita as I headed out the door for my early morning runs after the summer Olympics. In my head I thought of her as "Dita" and her name was a chant moving me forward when I got tired and wanted to slow down. In the summer of 2008, at thirty-eight years old, this Romanian mother became the oldest Olympic marathon champion in history. She wasn't expected to win. The night she won, my husband and I watched her run. Pumping her arms, her mouth set, she was determined, and it looked like she was barely breathing. With more than 10 miles to go, she broke away from the pack and left them grimacing in her shadow.

The morning after Dita's win was muggy. I left the house and told my family I'd be back soon.

"Just going for a quick run," I said. It had rained the night before and there were mud puddles along the greenway that I had to jump over. The sun was coming through the clouds and breaking them apart, making the sky a Lilly Pulitzer kind of pinky orange. I ran slowly because of the thick, wet air and when I began to lag and wanted to walk, I thought of Dita and kept going. I'd watched her run past Tiananmen Square and instead of my own marsh grass and pluff mud, I visualized Dita's foreign onlookers and China's brightly colored buildings. Like Dita, I pushed my legs harder and swung my arms faster. As I came around my last corner, I heard the crowds cheering inside the Bird's Nest and felt the desperation of the chase group behind me.

I started running when I was fifteen years old after I was diagnosed with Type 1 diabetes. When I asked my doctor if that meant I couldn't play sports (I'd been hoping for an excuse to miss field hockey practice), he laughed and told me exercise would help keep my blood sugars in check. So when the field hockey season ended, I started running. I preferred running alone because I didn't want to go with someone who might be faster or want to go farther; I liked my own steady pace. I didn't enjoy competition, and as a runner I didn't have to worry about missing the ball or sitting on the bench. There was no crowd watching, no one to cheer me on, and so I ran to the beat of my own steady breathing.

As the years passed, I began to call myself a runner. I bought running shoes from a real running store, learned how to properly stretch and cool down. I was happy to discover that running improved my blood sugars and decided it was time to enter my first race. I sent in money for a 5K, Race for the Cure, but didn't tell anyone. The morning of the race, as I neared the finish line, I pushed past my competition, my legs burning, and couldn't wait to race again.

Slowly, I began collecting race T-shirts and recognizing faces at local runs. When a fellow runner mentioned she was going to a Team in Training meeting, I decided to go along. By the next weekend, I found myself at six in the morning standing at the edge of a downtown lake with a group of strangers. Our plan was to run eight miles. I panicked as the group set off at a fast pace, worried that I was not ready. What if my blood sugar got low? What if I couldn't keep up? I didn't look like a runner; I was tall and had big feet that seemed to smack the pavement instead of springing from it like my friend Mary. As my friend moved ambitiously to the head of the pack, I found myself in the back. I didn't want to be in the back, so I kept my eyes on Mary and ran a little faster. By the time we reached our first water stop, I was solidly in the middle of the pack, breathing hard, my legs burning, but feeling strong.

Every week I drove to Mary's house and we ran from one end of the island and back. I carried a rolled-up dollar in my shorts to buy a Gatorade in case I got low, or a small bag of Skittles that always melted by the end of the run. When I was tired and wanted to stop and walk, I looked for Mary's legs tapping steadily along the trail in front of me, and that kept me going. Every Sunday from September to December, we met our group at the lake and ran farther than the week before.

By the time the marathon arrived, I stepped across the starting line confident that I would finish. Mary ran ahead of me, and I worked to maintain a steady pace alongside my aunt Sue, a veteran marathoner, who flew to Florida to run with me. With Sue and cheers from the crowd, I ran for four and a half hours, all the way to the finish line. I wore the medal around my neck all day, and when we flew home, I hobbled down the narrow aisle toward my seat on the airplane, surrounded by my family.

It's been twelve years since that day and now I'm back to running alone. Every morning, while my family sleeps, I run the same familiar 3-mile route. As a thirty-eight-year-old mother of three, I can no longer imagine running a marathon; it seems like a memory from another life. I tell myself that I don't have three free hours to spend on Sunday mornings running, and if I did, I would spend that time in other ways: wandering through the aisles of a bookstore, writing on my laptop in a coffee shop, or driving out to the beach and going for a short run along the sand.

But then I watched Dita run through the city of Beijing and something woke up inside me. Something told me it was time to race again. Dita's gritty ambition reminded me of how good it felt to race, and that being a mother didn't mean you couldn't compete.

On Thanksgiving morning, I left the rental house by the sea with my three sons and headed to the beach for the 5K/1-mile Turkey Trot family run. Instead of running shirts, there was a turkey mascot at the starting line and raffle tickets for apple pies. Leaving the smaller ones behind, I stood at the starting line next to my eight-year-old son. When they blew the whistle, we took off together. Will and I started slow, I carried his fleece when he got warm, and I listened when his breathing got heavy. At the half mile mark my son turned to head toward his own finish line, and I continued down the beach with the adults. I wanted to look back and watch my boy compete, but it was my turn now, so I picked up the pace. I could hear the voices of Mary, Sue and Dita cheering me on.

~Amy Stockwell Mercer

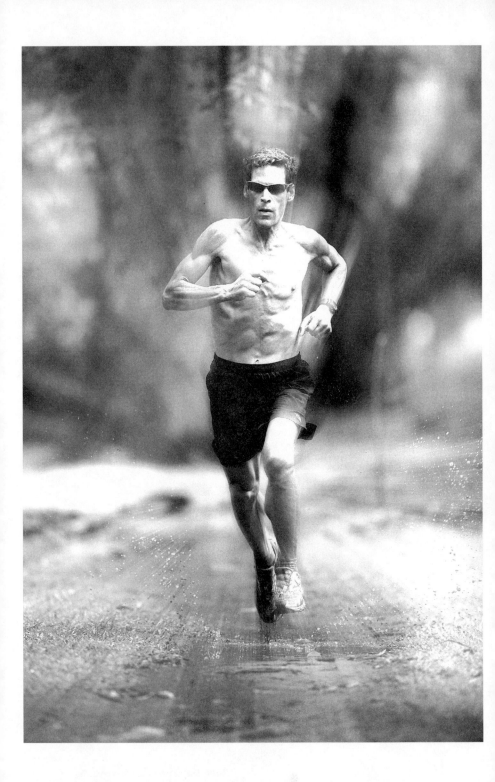

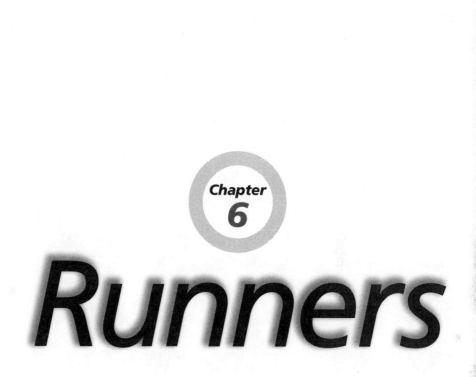

Runners

Chapter 6

Family Ties

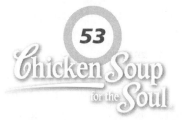

53

The Best Race of My Life

Fame is rot; daughters are the thing.
~James Matthew Barrie

I live for extreme adventures. The more intense, the more remote, the harsher, the better. I've raced and competed on all seven continents of the planet, twice over now, and have seen some of the most exotic places imaginable: the Gobi desert, Antarctica, Patagonia, the Dolomites, the Atacama desert, Namibia, to name a few. I've run hundreds of miles without rest in some of the most savage conditions the Earth has to offer. Once, I even ran 50 marathons, in all 50 states, in 50 straight days.

So when people ask me what my favorite race has been, my answer sometimes surprises them. It wasn't a hundred mile race through the mountains, it wasn't a six-day trek across the Sahara, it was a 10K (yep, that's a mere 6.2 miles). Allow me to explain why.

Beyond being an ultramarathoner, my first priority is always my family. They take precedence over all else. It's just who I am, it's how I'm hardwired. A proud father and husband, nothing is more important to me than my family.

With that said, I have never "pushed" running on my two children, fearing the proverbial parental backlash. If my kids, Alexandria, age nine, and Nicholas, age seven, wanted to run, that would be great. If not, that was their prerogative and I would love them regardless.

Neither of them had shown a particular interest in running. They'd accompanied me on many of my marathons and ultramarathons, so I knew they had been exposed to my antics from the day they were born. But there just didn't seem to be much of an interest in running on their behalf.

So you can imagine my shocked astonishment when Alexandria approached me two weeks before her tenth birthday and informed me that she wanted to run a 10K with me to celebrate the occasion. At first, I wasn't sure how to react. Was she doing this just to appease me? Was this something she really wanted to do for herself? My mind was awhirl with questions.

When the day came, she seemed excited as ever to take up the challenge. At ten years old, running 6.2 miles would not be easy. But she seemed genuinely interested in doing just that.

When the gun went off and the race began, she darted out at neck breaking speed. I knew such an approach was imprudent because one could only hold such an aggressive pace for a short duration and the toll it could take during the later stages of the race could prove disastrous. Still, I fought back my fatherly impulse to counsel her, bit my lip, and, frankly, did all that I could to keep up with her.

By the halfway point, her initial vigor had begun to taper. Running three miles at such a fast pace had left her nearly exhausted. As a father, it was tough to see my daughter so worn out when I could have advised her to slow down and take it easy in the first few miles to help preserve her energy.

Approaching the five-mile mark, the cumulative effects of the running along with the sheer number of minutes on her feet were really starting to show. She huffed and puffed and struggled to maintain her focus. Things were not looking good. I'd never seen her so exhausted before, and it hurt me. I couldn't allow this to continue.

Just as I was about to turn to her and tell her how incredibly proud I was of her for having the courage to have tried, and congratulate her for being able to run five miles, she turned to me and said, "Dad, I'm going to make it."

Never before have I seen such grit and determination to persevere in anyone, let alone a ten-year-old! She put her head down, let out an audible grunt, and charged into the abyss with unflinching resolve.

People along the course were in total disbelief, as was I. She was a woman on a mission, entirely focused on the task at hand, pumping her arms resiliently and thrusting her legs boldly forward with every stride. They cheered for her and applauded wildly as she bounded by.

Forget about me, I was a complete mess. I tried my best to choke back the tears, but finally gave in to my emotions. I was a sobbing child, huge tears running down both cheeks, completely unable to regain my composure no matter how hard I tried.

As we rounded that final corner and the end came into focus, she issued her final tear-wrenching dictum. "Daddy," she said. "Give me your hand. I want to hold it when we cross the finish together."

I did as she requested and we burst across that finish line as a team. People rushed over to her and began offering her aid and assistance. "I'm fine," she told them. "Really, I'm fine." To be honest, it was me who needed the help; I'd come completely unraveled. I've crossed deserts on foot, run single-handedly over high mountains, forged solo across raging rivers, but nothing had ever impacted me the way the sight of that little girl refusing to give up in the face of overwhelming adversity had. It was the most glorious moment of my life.

The memory of Alexandria and I crossing that finish line together has replayed beautifully in my mind on countless occasions. No matter how many trophies I earn, no matter how many records I set, no matter how many distinctions I have the good fortune of being bestowed upon me, nothing will ever top that moment.

When that final day beckons and I take my last earthly breath, her wonderful memory on that fateful day together will allow me to run off into the eternal sunset with an ever-enduring smile upon my face.

~Dean Karnazes

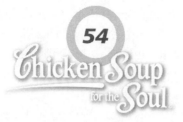

54

Running Home

There's nothing half so pleasant as coming home again.
~Margaret Elizabeth Sangster

I slowly tied the laces of my running shoes, imagining that he was doing the same. It was eleven hours ahead where he was stationed—although the distance felt much farther. The weather outside was overcast, a typical Western Washington morning. The clouds filling the sky and steady threat of precipitation were a stark contrast to the hot and dusty terrain he would navigate through. Our iPods played the same music, having been downloaded from the same computer several months earlier. We would breathe in the same broken pattern, running at the same speed, yet we'd be a world apart.

I stepped onto the sidewalk, pushing the jogging stroller that carried our toddler through the tree-lined street, passing homes filled with electronics, toys, and plentiful food. I wondered what he was looking at as he prepared for his workout. The pictures he'd sent home contained images of dust storms and dirt roads strewn with gravel. The homes were simple, the villages housed inside brick walls, with no decorative waterfalls or greenery. Children came out to greet the soldiers, begging in Arabic for candy, pens, and pencils. He was able to decipher what they asked, handing over all of the pens he carried in his uniform pocket.

I ran at a steady pace, breathing in the cool air, waiting for the endorphin rush which always accompanied my run. The only fear that lay ahead of me was the anticipation of the hills I'd embark upon during my exercise, while pushing a stroller. Neighbors waved as I ran past, nodding their heads while tending to their flower beds or gathering their morning newspaper. My older children had already departed on the school bus, where they were guaranteed a day of learning, fun, and safety. I calmly switched to a song with a more upbeat tempo, to push me through my morning run, as the tiredness and worry which consumed each day threatened to halt my workout.

I imagined him setting out on his run, along the dusty streets of the military base, in Western Iraq, during what was his second overseas deployment. He'd jog in the secure enclosure of a fenced-off installation, guarded by soldiers. There were no neighbors doing yard work or carefree kids leaving for school. The grade school children in the neighboring village walked along the gravel roads, if they were able to attend school at all. He ran in the secure enclosure to avoid the threat of hidden explosive devices and the stray bullets of insurgents, eager to hurt him if the opportunity arose. He ran outside cautiously, only if the dust sat close to the ground and the burn pits were not ablaze, to spare his lungs.

My heartbeat strengthened as I pushed the jogging stroller that carried our youngest daughter, to the rhythm of my movement. I wasn't prepared to say goodbye to my husband as he left for another twelve-month deployment. I'd found few things as heartwrenching as the looks of fear and confusion on the faces of our children in the months he'd been gone. I'd like to think I possessed a mountain of inner strength in the midst of fear that soldiers would arrive at my front door to deliver the news that my husband of twelve years had been killed in the line of duty. That, however, would be untrue—the fear was always there, in the back of my mind, from the moment I woke in the morning, through the nightmares in my sleep.

I pushed myself further, knowing that although my life was filled with unpredictable, chaotic, and overwhelming moments, running was something I still controlled. I wasn't the fastest runner, or the one with the most endurance, but I ran because I enjoyed it, because it gave me energy, and filled me with power. When I ran, I didn't feel the fear or loneliness—I rather felt strength, as though I was capable of handling the pressures of being his military wife, their single mother, and the person I wanted to be when I looked in the mirror at night.

I visualized my husband, winded as he continued his nightly run, wearing his standard physical training uniform, black shorts with a gray T-shirt. As his heart pulsed a steady beat, I recognized he was running for his life, to survive the rigors and dangers of war. He exercised to fend off the boredom that crept into his daily routine, to stave off the loneliness in the quiet hours of his night, and to forget the regret he carried with him over being so far away from his children when they cried for him. Although he was in Iraq—not running with me—he was running toward us, in an effort to come home. Amid the stifling hot weather, the soldiers in uniform, and care packages lovingly sent by priority mail, he was trying to cross the finish line of one of the longest races of his life.

As I rounded the corner onto our street, I felt his strength beside me, picturing the beads of sweat lining his forehead as his stride lengthened. Even half a world away, his presence was felt in our everyday lives, as though he were sitting with us at the dinner table or reading bedtime stories with the kids. I heard the sound of his laughter as we raced toward the house, challenging one another to finish first. My heart knew that while I ran alone, he was always with me in every step I took.

I looked at the flower beds in front of our house, where the tulips poked through the early spring ground, a reminder that he would return home in just a few months. Eventually, we would cross this finish line together—having survived another deployment. It was a race we'd always remember and look back on with both happy and painful memories, forever thankful for the life we've built together. We will continue to run beside one another, knowing that no matter the course, each race is worth the challenge.

~Melissa Blanco

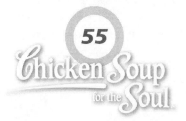

55

My Running Partner

Now bid me run, and I will strive with things impossible.
~William Shakespeare

In May of 1988, I started a new job and met Paul. He found many pretenses to come to my office, usually bringing an entertaining story or joke along with the ostensible reason for his visit. Six weeks later, at a Friday night gathering at a local pub, he finagled a seat across from me. In case I didn't already understand, he made his romantic interest perfectly clear. I enjoyed no similar interest in him, but something kept me from rejecting him completely. I settled on the old line, "Let's just be friends."

Undaunted, Paul continued the chats. He wanted to know all about me, including my running, which was peculiar since Paul made no attempt to exercise. His diet was unhealthy (high fat, few vegetables) and he smoked. He apparently wanted to show me that he was interested in everything about me, even the ways in which I was different from him.

During that same summer, another co-worker walked into my office with an application for a road race. He knew I ran but had never entered a race. Apparently he thought I should. I didn't consider myself an athlete, but the application refused to disappear. It lay there—taunting me. Three days later, I mailed it in.

After the race, as we were drinking Gatorade and eating bagels, I was shocked to hear my name called for second place in my age group. This was a first for me, someone who had never before done anything athletic.

From the shelf in my family room, the small award dared me to enter another race. I hoped to earn that heady feeling of achievement again.

By August, Paul's humor was melting my resistance. When I mentioned the first race in September, he said he wanted to go with me.

He became an enthusiastic supporter, getting up before dawn to tramp through cool, dewy fields to the start and wait with his camera at the finish. Six months later, we were living together. Within another year, we were engaged.

In 1992, I joined a marathon training program. After each run, Paul greeted me with coffee on the back porch, and eagerly listened to the morning's adventure. He lent encouragement during my first marathon, and met me at the finish to rejoice at my 4:28 time (considerably faster than the five hours I had hoped for). Occasionally, he even joined me on short runs, in spite of the fact that he still smoked.

A year later, he joined the marathon training program himself. The Sunday he ran 8 miles for the first time, he said it was much harder than he had expected. But since he had never run that far before, he thought maybe that's simply what 8 miles felt like. Besides, he had a persistent cold. Later that week, he also had a fever and decided to see a doctor.

Paul went to a nearby clinic, where he was diagnosed with pneumonia. When he went back for a follow-up visit, the doctor was disappointed that a dark area remained in one lung. Two weeks later, a bronchoscopy revealed a large, inoperable, malignant tumor. It wrapped around the trachea and right bronchial tube, partly closing it. No wonder Paul had difficulty running 8 miles. Paul declined chemotherapy, but began radiation therapy right away, which his oncologist said offered the greatest hope.

I had been more content than ever before — my kids were grown, I liked my job, I was in good health, and I had a loving fiancé. Now my future had been ripped out of my hands. I was unable to accept the bleak prognosis. There had to be help somewhere, and I intended to find it. I had little time for anything other than searching for alternative treatments, since traditional medicine offered little hope.

But in the midst of my search, Paul insisted I take the time to run. He said it was more important than ever for me to have that one bit of normalcy and the support of our running friends. He was right. They told me stories of courage and beating the odds, as well as giving us advice about several non-traditional therapies.

Even though the radiation therapy weakened him, Paul insisted on going with me in October to my first big city marathon—the Marine Corps Marathon in Washington, D.C. After we returned, his condition worsened. Even so, he insisted I keep running for both of us, which I did until the last month before he passed away.

After his death, grief paralyzed me. I could barely make it through a workday. I couldn't cook, I couldn't shop, and I certainly couldn't run.

Six weeks later, Sophie, a fellow runner, called and asked me to run with her the next Sunday morning. I made excuses, but she insisted.

Sophie knew just what to say while we ran. She reminded me that Paul wanted me to go on with my life, including my running. She suggested we meet in a few days for another run. I did. Running reminded me I was alive.

Running had been a thread throughout my relationship with Paul, and now it would have a role in easing my grief.

In November of that year, I ran the New York City Marathon in Paul's memory. He had so wanted to go with me to New York, to show me where he grew up, to show me the sights of Manhattan. Though he wasn't with me physically, I felt his presence every step of the way. I was sure I saw him in the crowds with his camera. I know he saw me cross the finish line. I even heard, "Way to go, Bet."

~Bettie Wailes

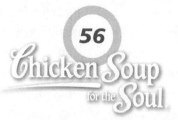

Recovered Memories

It's surprising how much of memory is built around things unnoticed at the time.

~Barbara Kingsolver

I'll always remember 1979 as the year Janine and I ran our last marathon together. Running tech, (technology, technique and training), was a far cry then from what it is today. Good running shoes were as rare as Spandex and just as expensive. Janine and I usually saved the good stuff for races, training in bargain-store sneakers and cut-off jeans, whatever we could fish out of the laundry basket.

Sunday runs had replaced Sunday mass for this fallen Catholic and Gatorade had become my holy water. I gulped it with salt tablets to replenish my electrolytes (whatever they were) and wolfed down plates of spaghetti before every big race. Carbohydrate loading was the mantra of the moment, the best and blessed buzz words of runners in the know. At least that's the way I remember it. After years of washing down my racing pasta with Chianti I had more than a few of my own buzzes going on, so who can know for sure?

Janine didn't enter her first marathon until 1975, a time when running's Dark Ages were just coming to an end. Our daughters might be shocked to learn that the Boston Marathon didn't lift its ban on women runners until 1972 and probably wouldn't have lifted it then if not for the negative publicity Beantown's event garnered a few years earlier when a race official-turned-bouncer tried to manhandle Kathrine Switzer off the course. Luckily, Switzer's boyfriend was running beside her and did a better job of manhandling the official. Kathrine finished the race, shaken but unbowed.

Like Switzer and her beau, Janine and I were running side by side in the '78 and '79 Maryland Marathon. Our times in both races were about three and a half hours, not too shabby for a married couple trying to sandwich daily training sessions between slices of sleep and full-time jobs.

Don't think I didn't catch your half-mumbled "so what?" or the thump of a forehead on the coffee table. This old writing teacher is savvy enough to recognize the sound of a reader nodding off mid-paragraph. But bear with me, pour yourself a cup of coffee and take a NoDoz if you feel the need. I promise you we're getting to the story's hook.

I'll grant you that if the ghost of Phidippides kept a ledger of every marathon ever run there'd likely be enough married couples running races together to fill a phone book. But don't go looking for Janine and me in that book because we won't be there.

We were married all right, just not to each other. Janine and I didn't even know each other then... and wouldn't for more than a quarter century.

She showed up in one of my writing classes a few years ago, umbrella in hand (to remind me it was raining outside) and wearing spike heels with her jeans (to remind me how French women dressed... did I mention Janine was born in France?). Until that moment I'd been the consummate pro who'd never forgotten a lecture. But now I found myself speechless for a moment, summoning the courage to pull a shopworn pick-up line out of mothballs, when Janine beat me to it.

"You look familiar," she said. "Do we know each other?"

We both knew it wasn't a pick-up line because we both had the feeling we'd seen each other before, not once but dozens of times. The nagging question was where?

That evening I noticed an old photograph gathering dust on my mantle. Framed in one of those clear plastic boxes popular in the seventies, the photo showed me nearing the finish line of the '78

Maryland Marathon. I picked up the frame and slid out the cardboard backing. Don't ask me why. I peeked inside. Behind the photograph was my sweat-stained race number and a folded edition of the *Baltimore Sun* with the race results. I was more than a little startled to find Janine's name just a few lines below mine on the finishers' list. Our times were less than 2 minutes apart.

Months later, over coffee at Starbucks, I told Janine of the list I'd found behind my photograph and how we'd competed side by side so long ago. She smiled and produced a photograph of her own, showing a group of runners training on one of the hilly roads winding through Maryland's Loch Raven Reservoir. I recognized the road immediately and why not? I'd run it hundreds of times. Janine was in the foreground of the photo, surrounded by an elite group of runners, including the great Olympic miler, Marty Liquori.

"Recognize anyone?" she asked.

"You must be kidding," I said, handing back the picture. "I know who Marty is."

"Recognize anyone else?"

"The woman looks familiar," I said, glancing at the photo. Janine wasn't buying into my sarcasm, so I looked again. I noticed a bearded figure in the background, wearing a threadbare green ski jacket. "I had a jacket just like that," I said, my chair beginning to resemble a dunce stool.

Now Janine and I understood why we'd looked so familiar to one another. We'd trained on the same roads and ran the same races for years, probably passed each other a hundred times. Yet we never said hello. Or maybe we did, just didn't remember.

A psychologist might call the sudden flood of "Janine" images coursing through my temporal lobes a case of recovered memory, while the cynic might call it wishful thinking. Maybe it was a little of both.

Eventually Janine divorced her husband and I separated from my wife. Our children are grown. These days we're living a *Nights in Rodanthe* kind of life on North Carolina's Barrier Islands, writing our books, collecting sea shells and feeding the gray foxes and feral cats.

My knees and I gave up running years ago but Janine still runs every day through the little village near our home. Although she's always been the better runner, Janine knows I can still catch her now and again.

If I'm on my bicycle.

~Mike Sackett

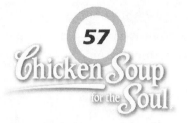

57

T-Shirt Tales

Be presidents of each other's fan clubs.
~Tony Heath

T he sky turned muted shades of pink as I jog-walked home from Sheri's. What a glorious way to begin the day. I desperately needed a break from the daily grind of job, family, and fixer-upper house projects. Running, my first serious athletic endeavor, would be that break.

I'd suggested that Hal and I run together evenings while our ten-year-old daughter watched the younger boys, begged even, but he wasn't interested. I was disappointed, hoping to recapture some of the closeness we'd had early in our marriage. But I called Sheri. Girlfriends will try anything.

"Tell me again why we're running?" she asked that first day as I coaxed her up a hill in our southwest Portland neighborhood.

"Because we want to be thin, healthy, and energetic."

"Why don't we just turn vegan? It's dark out here."

It was hard getting myself down our driveway or Sheri out her door some mornings. But we kept at it, blocks building into miles.

The day we ran three miles I bragged to Hal. "See? I am a runner. Want to join me now?"

"Runners always look like they're in pain."

I had to laugh, though I wished he'd said yes. I was in pain sometimes, but the slimmer, happier me was worth it.

"Ready for a new adventure?" I asked Sheri one morning. "There's a 10K out east of Gresham—the Turkey Trot."

"That's more than six miles."

"Think fall colors, free food, cool T-shirts. We're already up to four miles."

Sheri finally agreed when I offered a week of caramel mochas.

Hal was getting ready for work when I got home. "I want to do a race out in Gresham a week from Saturday," I told him.

"You're kidding, right?"

I could see his face in the bathroom mirror as he shaved. He looked surprised. What did he think I'd been doing all those mornings? "Maybe you and the kids could come cheer me on."

Hal kept right on shaving. "Sorry, Babe. Too much to do here."

I turned and left the bathroom, my excitement fading. Once he'd supported me in everything I did. Now he'd drawn some kind of line around his heart with me on the outside.

I channeled my disappointment into rigorous training, and the day of the Turkey Trot Sheri and I joined at least two hundred runners shedding sweat suits and stretching quads. I ran the first half of the race well, people lining the route cheering and clapping, my legs pumping like pistons, my spirits as high as the maples along the road. I wished Hal could see me. The next three miles I just kept moving, arms and legs aching, chest heaving. Sheri trotted beside me, red-faced and silent, except when she said she'd never run again. We were the last two runners on the course to cross the finish line.

"We did it!" I gave Sheri a sweaty hug.

When I got home I found Hal installing some shelves in the garage. "I finished," I bragged.

"That's great." He didn't even look up as he screwed down another shelf.

That line around his heart seriously hurt me. I didn't recover my good mood until I put on my Turkey Trot T-shirt. I wore that shirt proudly for days.

I ran through the winter, alone now because Sheri really had quit. My runs were my meditation, renewing mind and body.

I didn't ask Hal to join me, not wanting more rejection, but when the first crocus bloomed I got a yen to do another 10K, found out about the Rock Creek Run in farmlands west of Portland, and asked him to come with me to that. There would be baby calves and lambs. The kids would love it.

"I need to get the soil ready for the garden," he said. He was, in fact, thumbing through *Organic Gardening* magazine.

"I'll help when we get home. Please. It would be fun."

"For you, maybe."

"Could you do something, just once, because it's important to me?" Tears of frustration burned my eyes.

"Running's your thing, not mine." That line again.

My mind churned the morning I drove alone to Rock Creek. Was it just the running issue, or was my marriage on the rocks? But my spirits lifted as I ran past a herd of Holsteins, a tall, chestnut mare nose to nose with a shorter paint, and two bleating pygmy goats. Country smells filled the air.

I wished Hal and the kids could see it all.

When my thoughts turned to home, my steps slowed. My legs grew heavier. A runner passed me, and then another.

"Think of all the people sitting home reading their Sunday paper," an older man said as he jogged up alongside me. "They probably couldn't run a block."

"That's right. Thank you." My achievement and self-esteem were as tightly intertwined as my shoelaces. I picked up my pace and was still smiling when I crossed the finish line.

When I arrived home, Hal was rototilling the garden. I wanted to say, "Hey, I finished. And I wasn't last." But I just went in the house and drew a warm bath, not up to being hurt again. Afterward I put on my Rock Creek 10K T-shirt. I even wore it to bed.

I felt ready for a bigger challenge. "I want to do the Cascade Runoff," I told Hal one evening just before bed. "It's a 15K. Will you watch the kids?" I didn't ask him to go, and of course he didn't offer.

"You seriously think you can go the distance?" he asked.

I bristled. "You haven't even seen me run."

"Just trying to have a conversation." He climbed in bed and took a book from his nightstand.

A conversation? When had he shown any interest in my running? I missed the partner I'd married.

I channeled my heartache into training and felt confident the morning of the race, although sadness welled in me when I saw some of the runners at the start surrounded by their families.

We started out along the Willamette River, warm sunlight dancing on the water. High on endorphins, I ran mile after mile, gulping water at the way stations, and raising my arms in thanks when a group of volunteers offered to splash us with hoses. In the eighth mile, pain began shooting through my right knee, and my breath came in gasps. But in the ninth mile, when I turned a corner, I saw, ahead just another two blocks, a banner emblazoned with the words "Finish Line." I'd nearly done it.

Then, one block from the banner, I stopped and bent double, hands on knees, chest constricted, legs cramping. I couldn't run another step. Not for any amount of money, not to prove anything to Hal or myself, not even for chocolate. Had anyone before run the first nine miles of the Cascade Runoff, and then simply quit? Forget the half marathon. Forget the marathon. Forget personal bests, country sights, and weight loss. This must be what it felt like to die.

As I pushed damp hair from my eyes, I glanced across the street. Hal and my three children waved madly. "You can do it," Hal shouted.

He'd come! A burst of adrenaline pumped through my veins. I shot across the finish line and into the arms of my family. I knew Hal had crossed his own line the way our eyes met and held. None of my fantasies about running had included Hal and me locked in this moment of mutual appreciation, perhaps entering a better phase of our relationship. Where could I find a T-shirt that said, "My husband rocks?"

~Samantha Ducloux Waltz

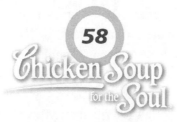

58

Cosmic Engineering

Maybe men and women aren't from different planets.... Maybe we live a lot closer to each other. Perhaps, dare I even say it, in the same zip code.
~Sarah Jessica Parker

hree schools in two states before third grade—it hadn't been easy for my eight-year-old daughter, Heather. I'd dragged her from the asphalt jungles of Southern California to the wilds of Northern Idaho. The students at the new school hadn't been very welcoming, and then even her "friends" turned on her.

All this time I was going through a lot of stress at work and in life. Changing jobs, company problems, layoffs, reduced pay, long hours and a long commute got me focused too much on myself and not enough on Heather's needs. She was growing up, facing challenges I wasn't really aware of and I was losing contact with my precious little girl. I sensed she was unhappy, but I didn't really understand her anymore. I wondered what had gotten into her. She seemed moody... distant.

You may have heard of *Men Are From Mars, Women Are From Venus.* I began to wonder if children are from Pluto! (This was back in 1999 when far-away Pluto was still universally recognized as a planet.)

But when Heather told me about something called "Bloomsday" practice she was doing at school, she got my attention. My little daughter was in training for a 12K race to be held that spring across the state line in Spokane, Washington. Every year, 50,000 people gather in Spokane to run or walk the approximately 7.5 miles for the glory of receiving a Bloomsday T-shirt!

I've been a jogger for years—it's about the only exercise I get with all that time behind the wheel and behind a desk. It may not have given me a runner's high, but it has always been a nice way to ease into the day. So when Heather mentioned Bloomsday, I was in! I thought it would be a great way to spend some time together and share this positive hobby.

I hadn't entered a race since my school track days. I had no illusions about winning—I still had the cinders in my shoulder from my first race wearing cleats, when I beat my best 400-meter time and then tripped on the final curve of the 800-meters. Besides, I needed to stay with Heather, and her legs were only half as long as mine. I didn't want to lose her in that crush of humanity!

Over the months before Bloomsday we had the chance to train together a few times—not nearly as many as we wanted because of sickness, business trips and a busy life. But I'll always treasure those times, as running, walking and talking about the things on her mind gave me a much greater grasp of what things were like on Pluto.

On the day of the race itself, Heather and I headed out early, caught the shuttle bus from an outlying mall and made our way through the crowd to a starting position far back in the pack.

Heather was shocked and dismayed that even after the race officially started, we weren't able to go anywhere! When our part of the crowd finally started moving, it wasn't even at a walking pace—we were waddling more like penguins. Slowly it picked up to a walk, and then we found an opening and began to jog.

It was a beautiful day, and we were doing this together! Truth be told, I wasn't that interested in getting to the finish line. I wished it could go on forever. I hadn't really had time to study the route, so I honestly couldn't tell how far we had gone or how much we had left. So since neither of us had run a race at this distance, I suggested we conserve our energy and walk for a while. Sooner than I expected, off in the distance I thought I saw hints of the finish line.

Heather couldn't believe that all the people around us were still walking if we were so close to the end! She took off like a bullet! I could see that all her training, her young legs and our energy conservation had paid off, but I feared I would lose her! I never overcame her head start, and she beat me handily across the line. I lost the race, but thankfully I didn't lose her!

We grabbed our T-shirts—the green ones Heather said looked like they had squirts of ketchup, mustard and grape jelly on them! Someone was selling cotton candy, and Heather's eyes lit up. Just this once, I thought. It was a special day.

Epilogue:

Recently I pulled that old Bloomsday T-shirt from the bottom of the drawer. It still fits, and it brings back great memories. Heather's little shirt is long gone—that was more than half her life ago—but mine brings back memories for this amazing high school senior too.

"Want to go running, Dad?" she asks. We take off at a leisurely jog through our tree-lined neighborhood in Ohio, talking about the differences between men and women (she's read the Mars/Venus book too). She tells me that men are always trying to fix things, instead of just listening. I take the hint and listen contentedly.

The conversation drifts to calculus, college choices and cotton candy. She still remembers that after all these years. "I thought it was pretty special just hanging out with my daddy," she says.

I'll never forget Bloomsday either. We didn't set any speed records. But still I think we did a little cosmic engineering—moving Mars and Pluto just a little closer to each other.

~R. Mike Bennett

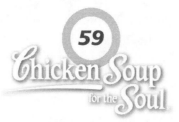

59

Extreme Corps Marathon and Stars

Running is the greatest metaphor for life,
because you get out of it what you put into it.
~Oprah Winfrey

"I'm running the Marine Corps Marathon!" my husband announced at dinner.

I shot back, "No, you're not!"

Mark, my husband of eighteen years, snapped back, "Oh, yes, I am and that's final!" He spoke like a Marine Corps drill sergeant.

Our family had barely recovered from Mark's last attempt at a marathon, which took months of preparation. The night before each run, I strategically placed nourishment along the course: bottles of Gatorade hidden behind telephone poles; PowerBars stored underneath rocks; and water bottles perched alongside road signs—all in an effort to get my husband to his next "extreme" goal.

Mark's recent announcement came just as we sat down to dinner. Jon, our younger son, folded his hands tightly and prayed, "Dear God, please help Daddy win this time!" He heaved a sigh of relief and shoved his spoon into the bowl of mashed potatoes.

Why was I dragging my feet? Didn't I know how important this was to my husband—sort of a mile marker before he turned forty? But it was his goal—not mine—and now we were all going to pay the extreme price in training for the event.

Mark explained that this time would be different: Oprah Winfrey was running the Marine Corps Marathon with him. My eyes lit up. A chance to see Oprah run… that was worth it! Suddenly the whole idea of a marathon changed. No longer did I see tedious training runs before the big event; I saw an opportunity to rub elbows with a star. Could it be that I was actually going to get an up close and personal look at one of my favorite television celebrities?

For days—no weeks—we marked red "X's" on the calendar as each run brought us one "step" closer to the Marine Corps Marathon (and Oprah Winfrey!).

Jon—who was seven years old at the time—asked, "Is Daddy really going to run with O-pah?"

I guess he heard me talk more about the "star" than his dad's participation in the event.

Carefully forming my words, I said, "No, your dad will be running in the same race with Oprah, but they won't be running together. Do you understand?"

Jon nodded his head "yes" and ran upstairs to play video games.

The following week, Mark continued with the planned schedule for the 20-mile run (the final "leg" of the journey before the actual event). I placed nourishment under rocks; Gatorade behind lamp posts, and once again hid behind trees to make sure no one took the precious contents before Mark could retrieve them. Twenty miles would serve as the last endurance test before the race.

The morning of the marathon, we packed up the car and hit the Capital Beltway before 5:00 AM for the three-hour drive into Washington, D.C., where the race was being held. There were legions of cars, newspaper reporters, and a mammoth entourage for Oprah.

What we hadn't planned on and what we couldn't have anticipated was the uncooperative weather. A slight chance of rain turned into a torrential downpour. We sloshed through inches of mud—on the once grassy turf—as we waited in long lines to register. We had one pink umbrella, a soggy blanket (reserved for Mark), and an already drenched rain poncho (size extra small). Mark positioned himself with the other runners while we waited for the "star" to appear.

Jon tugged on my coat and asked, "Mom, can we go home now? I'm tired!" I didn't have the heart to tell him that the race hadn't even started yet!

I hugged him tightly and said, "No, honey, we came to see your daddy run in the big race—remember?"

"Nuh-ah, you came to see O-pah!" he shouted defiantly and scooted away.

No sooner had the words left his mouth when I caught a glimpse of Oprah exiting her trailer, along with her trainer. I jockeyed for position to snap a picture, but it was futile. The runners merged into one big blur for the start of the race.

I stood on a tree stump to get a better view and caught a glimpse of Mark near the middle third of the formation. He was shivering. He stood for two hours in typhoon-like conditions with no protection except for a pair of flimsy running shorts and a T-shirt. Before I could make my way to Mark to tell him it was okay to turn back, the shot was fired to signal the beginning of the race.

We cheered on every wet, soggy, and mud-drenched runner as they passed by—giving shouts of praise, "Great job... keep going... don't give up!"

As the runners entered the first half of the race, we headed for the bridge closest to the finish line hoping to catch a glimpse of the star runner—Oprah—and her entourage. My older son, Jeremy, grabbed onto my soggy coat sleeve and shouted, "Mom, there she is—there's Oprah!"

I couldn't believe it. My husband was running alongside Oprah and they were talking!

Jon turned to me and said, "Mom, I thought you said Daddy wasn't running with O-pah?"

I was shocked—stunned really!

"What's he saying?" Jon asked.

"I'm not sure, but I think we'll find out later," I said.

Soaked and drenched, Mark made his way to the 20-mile mark. We shouted as he passed by, "You're almost there... don't give up!"

And then suddenly Mark turned and started running off course and into the crowd.

"No, Mark, you're going the wrong way… go back, go back!" But he kept running toward us—shaking his head—signaling defeat.

"Don't give up… you're almost there!" I screamed. I pointed to the street and waved my hands, "Go back!"

Jon clutched my raincoat and whispered, "Mom, I think Daddy's lost!"

"No, honey, he's just confused; he'll be fine," I countered.

It was no use. Mark had surrendered. No amount of shouting was going to change the outcome. Mark stared right through me—glassy-eyed and dazed. That's when I realized he was in a state of hypothermia. His legs cramped up and finally gave out underneath him.

A wounded heart is so much more difficult to heal than a blister on the foot. We watched as Oprah crossed the finish line and the shouts of glory rippled through the crowd—as if for a soldier coming home from war.

We gathered up our rain-soaked blankets and headed for the car. "Sorry, guys. I disappointed you," Mark said in defeat.

"No, Daddy, you won!" Jon shouted.

Jon pointed to the set of dog tags that Mark wore around his neck for security purposes. On one side were the words "Never Give Up" and on the other side was our cell phone number in case of an emergency. In Jon's eyes, his daddy had won the race!

My eyes were brimming with tears as Jon hugged Mark. Tears fell in a steady stream as I melted into the arms of my wounded "soldier." I took the dog tags from around Mark's neck and clutched them in my hand.

Jon grinned broadly, and with his green eyes shining, he said, "Daddy's a star, right Mom?"

"Yes, Jon, you're absolutely right—an extreme star!"

The human spirit is an amazing thing—especially in the heart of a runner. Mark never surrendered to defeat. Three weeks later, he ran the Harrisburg Marathon in Pennsylvania in 4 hours and 17 minutes.

It wasn't the "Marine Corps Marathon" that he had hoped for, but he did it—he never gave up. And in one little boy's eyes, he was already a winner!

~Connie K. Pombo

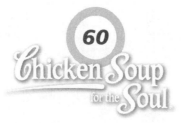

60

Saints at the Races

Endurance is not just the ability to bear a hard thing, but to turn it into glory.
~William Barclay

I want to draw attention to a group of endurance individuals who serve without honors, thanks or awards, and yet are highly deserving of canonization. These individuals are the family and crew of ultrarunners.

My husband Bob began his ultrarunning life in 1979 at a 50-mile race in Illinois. The following year he ran in a 100-mile race in California, and each year after that my three children and I have driven him around the United States from one ultrarun to the next. We are part of an elite group called the runners' "crew."

Crewing might seem like an easy job—drive around the race course meeting your runner at predetermined places, so that you can feed and encourage him and give him a change of clothes if needed. Piece of cake, right?

Let me give you a composite day in the life of my husband's crew.

The morning of the race starts very early, like at 3:00 AM. The 4:00 AM race start leaves no room for lagging children. At the start line I am encouraging my husband and listening to the moans of three tired, hungry, unhappy children. Who can blame them?

At the start line the gun goes off and the runners head off into the dark for 100 miles of grueling mountain terrain. Now my ultra begins. Get the children loaded into the van, and find a place open this early so that they can have a hot meal, the last one for the next thirty hours.

I check the map, given to me at the pre-race meeting, for the location of the first checkpoint. The sun has not yet risen above the horizon so seeing the turn-off roads is difficult. I try to keep my frustration level down as I turn around our full size van, which is not easy, and head back to the road I missed.

I park four blocks from the first checkpoint because of all the cars from crews that are already there. I strap my youngest child into his stroller and hand my daughter the folding chair and two of several gym bags that we will take. I attach the other gym bag to the stroller. My older son holds one handle of the cooler and I the other handle. One last check of the van to be sure we have not forgotten anything. We look like a caravan minus the camel.

The kids help me set up our mini-aid station. Now it is time to relax and wait. Okay, I entertain three children while we wait.

The kids spot their dad. The rhythm of the dance begins. Food is given, drinks are prepared, is it diluted Coke or Gatorade this time? Refill the water bottles. Take the cold weather gear that he wore early this morning; he won't need this again until evening. Fill his pack with a variety of snacks to fuel him until the next checkpoint. We kiss him goodbye.

I sigh. One down, many more to go. Repack the bags, put my youngest in the stroller, hand the chair to my daughter, distribute packs and share the carrying of the cooler with my son. This is repeated over and over.

I feed Bob information about his time at each aid station. He has to make cutoff times or he will be pulled from the race. This information is as important to him as the food I provide.

As the day wears on, my children and I are wearing down. Entertainment is hard to come by for young children in the middle of nowhere.

Darkness will be upon us in two hours. I need to think ahead. Bob will need warm clothing, a headlamp, and a flashlight, and I will need a flashlight too. "Don't forget anything," I chant to myself.

Bob arrives with wet shoes. He sits in the chair. I remove his shoes and roll the wet socks off. I dry his blistered, swollen feet. He will be heading into darkness and cold so I insist that he put his tights on. He will carry the long sleeve shirt, jacket, hat and gloves that I tie around him. It seems silly to take these things now but the cold of night will be on him before I see him again. Hypothermia is a real danger in these races. The kids have been handing their dad bananas, yogurt, raisins, peanut butter and jelly sandwiches and anything else that is in the cooler. He takes what he needs. Water bottles are refilled, his pack is resupplied with snacks. His headlamp is put in his pack and a flashlight is in his hand.

Each time I see my husband I am analyzing him. The medical checkpoints in the race evaluate the runners but there are things I watch for too. Is his gait different? His back might be hurting. I hand him Advil. Is he limping? A different pair of shoes may help.

At 75 miles my husband is in a stupor. I must do his thinking for him. He doesn't know what he needs or even what direction to go out of the aid station.

When he wants to quit I push him to his feet and tell him to go, I know he can do this. We live in Colorado but Bob suffers from altitude sickness, so if it hits him I have to stand with him and let him know it is okay to quit. I don't want him airlifted out because we overrode wisdom.

It is dark and my children are asleep in the van, I recline my seat and cover myself with a blanket. I don't sleep well. I am parked at the place that Bob will be passing; I don't have to wake my children.

Bob has been running and walking for more than twenty-six hours and the light of dawn is making its glorious appearance in the sky. I have had two very short naps.

We see Bob one last time before the finish line. The cut off time is thirty hours. He's going to make it. We give him a hug and kiss and tell him we'll see him at the finish.

At the finish area I take only my camera from the van.

In the distance I recognize Bob and a smile of relief spreads over my face. We are at the finish line cheering him across.

When Bob crosses that line my children and I are a part of his victory, but no one will give us a finisher medal, belt buckle, or certificate.

If a crew does its job well, all the runner has to think about is putting one foot in front of the other, over and over. We have done our job well.

In 2009, our thirty-five-year-old daughter, the one who had carried the chair for her father years before, followed in his steps and completed the Leadville 100-miler. Her dad, husband, friends and I were her crew. Coleen is 4'11" and less than one hundred pounds of grit.

The legacy continues.

~Diane Shaw

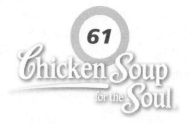

Marathon Mom

We are different, in essence, from other men. If you want to win something,
run 100 meters. If you want to experience something, run a marathon.
~Emil Zatopek

In 1980, when my children were old enough to stay alone for a few minutes, but young enough that it had to be only a few, I decided to make a dash to the store. I was thirty-four and breathlessly shocked that I couldn't run two blocks without stopping. It was at that moment I was humiliated enough to take up jogging. We lived near a park and the trek from my house around the park and back was a mile and a half. Day after day I ran the course until I could do it without stopping. I was a runner! Unfortunately I was soon an injured runner with no idea how to stop the pains in my shins, but I did know who to ask. Twice a day I would see a fellow run past my house. I knew he lived in the white house right across from the park. He seemed to run a little more than I did, so I figured he'd know what to do. I knocked on the door and the guy I'd seen running so often answered. He introduced himself as Garry and listened while I told him I was a runner (I actually said that) and asked if he knew anything about running injuries. He gave me lots of advice and suggested I go to a running store and replace my little tennis shoes with something better.

At the store I mentioned my neighbor and was treated like royalty. The clerk explained that the guy I'd been talking to was Garry Bjorklund, the Olympic runner, and didn't I know who he was? I knew enough to be totally embarrassed that I'd called myself a runner in his presence and resolved then and there to actually become one.

So I trained. Every day I ran a 5-mile loop, usually around 5:00 AM before my husband and kids woke up, and every day I would meet Bjorklund and a friend heading out as I was coming home. They always encouraged me, and I always picked up the pace.

In the fall of 1981, after a summer of intense training, I ran the City of Lakes Marathon. In order to get a T-shirt, you had to finish in less than four hours. I know it's shocking, but in those days, there were no bags of treats, medals, prizes, and news coverage. There were just some time officials, awards for the top finishers, and a T-shirt for finishing in under four hours. I finished the grueling 26.2 miles in about 4 hours and 20 minutes, which might very well have been last place. Most everyone had gone home except a wonderful volunteer who vowed to stay until the last person finished. But I was too late for the shirt.

I went home that day, thrilled to have run my first marathon but devastated that I had nothing to show for it. My kids made me tinfoil medals and when they hung them around my neck, I started to cry. I think I was still crying when the doorbell rang and there stood Bjorklund. "You're the one who deserves this," he said, and handed me a marathon shirt.

The Twin Cities Marathon replaced the City of Lakes Marathon in 1982 and instead of circling two lakes four times, it now winds around those lakes and continues on the scenic parkways and river roads of Minneapolis and Saint Paul. Thousands of supportive volunteers and hundreds of thousands of spectators with boom boxes blaring the theme from *Rocky* line the route to cheer on the more than eight thousand runners. It all ends up in front of the Capitol with great fanfare, copious amounts of food, medals for finishers, and, of course, the coveted T-shirt.

Marathons have come a long way since 1981, but they are still 26.2 miles. It has been twenty-five years since I ran that first marathon, twenty-five years since Bjorklund, a young man who'd won marathons, been an Olympian, and still holds the State high school boys' cross country 1600-meter record came to my house and handed me a shirt.

My own son, the tinfoil medal maker, and his sister are adults now, running their own marathons. In fact my son just qualified for Boston and last week called and said, "How about lacing up your running shoes again Mom, for me. Because you're a sixty-year-old woman, if you run a 4:30 marathon you'll qualify for Boston too! What do you say we go together?" Who can resist an offer like that? Time to get out that threadbare T-shirt and hit the road again!

~Bonnie West

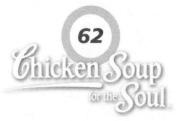

62

Sharing More Than a Jog

Movement is a medicine for creating change
in a person's physical, emotional, and mental states.
~Carol Welch

My dad had invited me to go running with him, and I was scared to death.

Dad and I have a somewhat colorful history. He's a long-time, binge alcoholic, so I entered a tumultuous home life at birth. There was fear, drama, and a time or two when the entire county's police force seemingly converged on our house. Growing up, I had a hard time figuring out exactly what to think of my father. Eventually he disappeared from our home life and I didn't have to think about him much for more than a year.

Visitation started toward the end of my elementary years, with me being the last of the children to submit to the court's order. I had a hard time seeing him as human. My mother fueled this by filling me with disturbing stories about him.

At the time of the running invitation, I was living more than a thousand miles away from him with a family of my own. He and his girlfriend were visiting for a week—one of the longest amounts of time I had spent with my father since my early childhood.

Running had been the focus of my dad's life since he was a teenager. I had run periodically throughout life, but inconsistently. Recently I had started running again, but only about three miles per day. Since my dad had run about one race per week for more than forty-five years, it would be a stretch to call me a chip off the old block.

During his visit, my dad and I were running separately each morning, and my dad was building up to asking me to join him. I pretended to miss the hints. Finally he said, "Erin, since we're both running, we should run together sometime." I was noncommittal—saying something about being slow and unsure of timing.

I was terrified that I would disappoint him. Why was I so concerned about impressing him, since he didn't exactly merit the "Father of the Year" award? He was a perfectionist—and he was my dad. I wanted him to be proud of his little girl, regardless of what kind of father he had been in those early years.

Saturday night he shocked me by asking, "So when is church tomorrow?" My self-proclaimed agnostic father took the initiative to attend church with us, rather than us inviting him.

I answered, "8:30."

"I'll be ready by then," he said. "I can probably even get my run in beforehand."

Sure enough, my father was standing next to me in a balcony pew Sunday morning. It was moving and surreal to have my father hold a hymnal with me and sing the words of "Victory in Jesus" aloud. Jesus is the center of my life, as running is the center of my dad's.

That whole day I fought an inner battle regarding our potential running date. I wanted to say yes, but I was petrified. That night I left a note for him: "If you hear me up by 6:20, plan on running together."

Sleepless that night, I could think of nothing but running with my dad. I prayed, "Lord, is there value in this?" The answer came quickly, "He sang 'Victory in Jesus' with you. If he can do that for you, you can run with him." I awakened well before 6:20.

We headed outside on that brisk November morning. "You lead," he said. "I'll follow your pace. Just do what's comfortable."

I took a deep breath and ran. He actually fell behind and then quickly caught up. "You run a faster pace than I expected," he said. That gave me the boost I needed. I continued my pace throughout our 2.5-mile or so jog. We talked a little on the run. I pointed out places where running stories I had shared with him had occurred in the past. He gave me tips without being at all intimidating.

I thanked God for giving me the courage to share my morning jog with the dad I was learning to understand. We both received a great gift. My dad shared the most important part of his life with one of the people he most loved in the world. And I experienced one of the tenderest moments I had ever had with him.

As we approached the end of our run, he said, "I'm impressed." I couldn't believe my ears, nor how much those words meant to me. He thanked me for running with him and said, "That was really special. I've never run with one of my daughters before." He said he would run farther after dropping me off. As we reached my home, he took my hand, squeezed it, and I watched as he ran on down the road.

~Erin Liddell

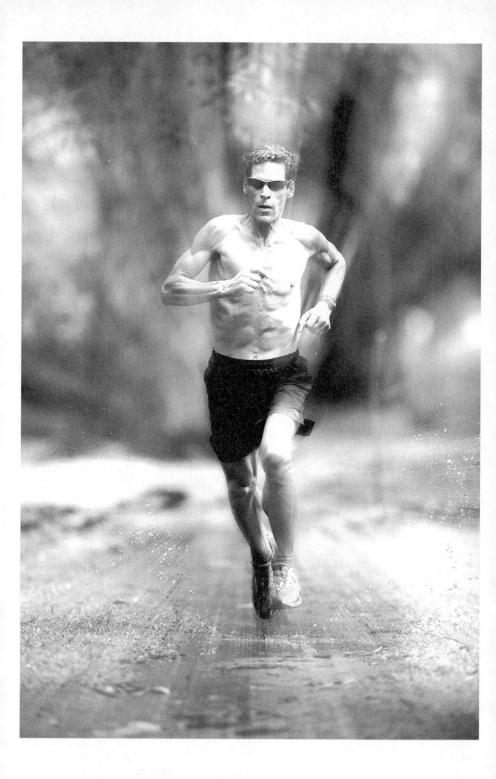

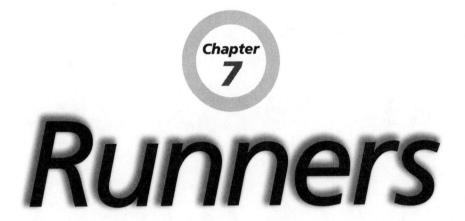

Runners

A Step at a Time

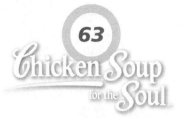

63

Finding Inspiration in Each Other

The best angle from which to approach any problem is the try-angle.
~Author Unknown

I took a long, hard look in the mirror at age thirty-one and faced a harsh reality. I definitely was not the same person I had been ten years earlier. The subtle changes that had occurred gradually over the years suddenly seemed drastic and the numbers on the bathroom scale emphasized my physical decline.

In 1980, while on work furlough during an economic downturn, I used the time off to catch up on projects around the house. One day, I was painting my garage when I noticed a woman running past. She was obese and was wearing a bulky, gray sweat suit, which reminded me of the one Rocky wore while getting in shape for his big fight in the first movie.

The next time the woman ran past my house, I glanced at my watch and then kept an eye out for her return. To my amazement, she jogged by nearly 90 minutes later. I thought she must be in better shape than she looked. This woman's determination made a lasting impression on me.

Another nudge was provided by an article in a health magazine, which said the lifestyle you settle into in your thirties is how you'll most likely live out the remainder of your life. For me, that was a scary prospect.

At the time, I was a parent volunteer at my daughter's elementary school. One of my first assignments was to chaperone a "Jump Rope for Heart" fundraiser. The children jumped rope for as long as they could to collect pledges for total minutes jumped.

I remember being especially impressed by one kid who jumped for more than an hour, proving that he was in great shape. At that point in my life, exercising for an hour seemed impossible. I tried jumping rope at the event and was embarrassed by how few minutes I could keep going. I bought one of the jump ropes, took it home and began my leap of faith into the exercise realm.

While helping in the school's pool several weeks later, the physical education teacher, Mr. Wondergem, asked if I had lost weight. My weight had crept up to 196 pounds at one point, but by then I had gotten down to the low 160s. I told him that I had lost weight and that I also planned to take up running now that I was no longer out of breath when I climbed a single flight of stairs.

Mr. W. suggested I read *Runner's World* magazine to get some running tips. The issue I picked up featured "How to Run Your First Marathon" and I was enthralled with the idea. Amby Burfoot, winner of the 1968 Boston Marathon, wrote the article, which was accompanied by a training chart with daily mileage requirements alternating with rest days. It all seemed so simple.

On my 32nd birthday, inspired by that obese woman jogging past my house, and armed with a training plan, I took my first steps as a runner. My initial goal was to run two miles. After only two blocks, I was forced to abandon the quest. I limped home and pondered my fate.

The following morning, I told my wife Gail I didn't think I would run that day because I hurt all over. She agreed that resting was probably a good idea. But then I asked, "Well, what will prevent me from saying the same thing the next day or the next?" I knew if I was going to reach my two-mile goal, it had to be a total commitment.

On my second outing, with each step more painful than the one before, my goal was simply to run a little farther than the previous day. As I continued training, I learned that I could go farther by taking walking breaks when it simply hurt too much to keep running.

Eventually, the walking breaks became less frequent and the small milestones of going farther each day helped me accomplish my bigger goal of running an entire two miles.

The next time Mr. W. remarked on my weight loss, my running mileage had increased and my weight was down to the 150s. He wondered how I had lost the weight so quickly. I told him I had followed his advice and read *Runner's World* and that I was following a marathon training plan. "You can't, Roy! You have to run a 2-mile race or a 5K or 10K before running a marathon," Mr. W. said.

Those were not the words of encouragement I was expecting. I had so often heard, from the time I was a little boy through adulthood, "You can't, Roy." It was time for the negativity to stop. I was determined to change those three discouraging words "You can't Roy" into "You can try!" Shifting a few letters changed my entire frame of mind.

In 1981, ten months after those painful first steps, I ran my first marathon. I was accompanied much of the way by a man who told jokes throughout the run, which made the time pass quickly. I had never run with anyone before that marathon and starting the race with 700 other runners was amazing. My time was 3 hours and 16 minutes and I enjoyed every step. I couldn't wait to tell Mr. W. about my accomplishment and let him know that he should never tell anyone they can't, but rather that they should TRY!

Before the marathon, I told Gail I was just going to run one race to see if I liked it. Man, did I like it! I ran fourteen more races that year and began training for my second marathon with a goal of qualifying for the Boston Marathon.

One day while on a training run on the country roads, a car pulled up and the gray-sweats lady, who never seemed to lose any weight despite all her running, offered me a ride. I declined, explaining that I was training for a marathon. She asked if I knew how far that was and after replying that I had already run a marathon, she drove off.

The next day, as I laced up my running shoes on my back porch, the woman ran by. I caught up to her and ran alongside and I asked her how far she ran each day. She told me she ran to the McDonald's to drink coffee and read the newspaper!

Fifteen years later I ran into the same woman, who was now much slimmer. "You don't remember me, do you?" she asked smiling. After looking into her eyes, I replied, "You used to be that obese lady who ran by my house!"

She had inspired me and I, in turn, had inspired her.

~Roy Pirrung

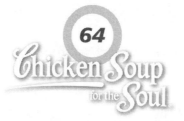

Running with the Wolf Pack

I hated every minute of training, but I said, "Don't quit. Suffer now and live the rest of your life as a champion."
~Muhammad Ali

I didn't get a chance to voice my opinion about running when I joined the Women's Army Corps. When "Aunt Sam" yelled "Double-time, march," off we went in a cloud of dust—no matter if our feet were blistered and our lungs felt ready to pop. Basic training is serious stuff. We'd run at 5 AM or at dusk—whenever they said, wherever they said.

I'd never run in my life, save for a few laps around my high school gym. I was a true tenderfoot. The first couple of days, our platoon practiced on an oval track, but soon we were running over steep hills, across sandy beaches, along winding paths. We would have run into the ocean had the drill sergeant pointed us in that direction but (luckily) she never happened to think of it.

Did we actually want to run? No! At the outset, most of us would have voted not to run at the crack of dawn, but to stay in our bunks for a little more shut-eye. We complained, we grimaced, we cussed. It wasn't as though we ever did anything when we got to our destination. We'd simply loop around and run back to where we'd started.

By the third week of training, we found our rhythm. We got in step and stayed in step, singing and clapping. The adventure of running as a team somehow made it seem easier. Whereas at the outset a mile seemed a sheer impossibility, soon we were chalking up three or more miles in a single stretch and hardly complaining. Our attitude had changed drastically.

No matter how exhausted we became, one thing was for sure — we never gave up. As distances increased, we became a crazed pack of wild wolves, fifty females strong, charging along together, pushing ourselves to limits we'd never even imagined. There was another hidden motivation to keep us on our feet. When we weren't running, we were stuck in the barracks either scrubbing (a floor, a toilet, a hallway) or polishing (shoes, boots, anything metal), so running had distinct advantages.

We never ran indoors. No matter if we would encounter sheets of rain, blinding sandstorms or even late snow flurries, we'd be outside in the fresh air — left, right, left, right — so many hundreds of thousands of steps you couldn't keep count. Running in our pack had become our way of life.

As all things do, our eight weeks of basic training drew to a close and it was time for fifty fast friends to part ways. Some would be shipped off to Korea, others to bases around the U.S., many of us to Europe.

The night before our graduation from basic training, we sat in a circle, our feet soaking in buckets of hot water. We laughed about how inept we'd been those first few days — how slow, how clumsy. It seemed a lifetime ago. At our graduation ceremony, we marched around the parade field at a normal walking pace. In our hearts we knew we were a wolf pack of strong women warriors — ready to run, run, run up against anything that dared to get in our way.

~Roberta Beach Jacobson

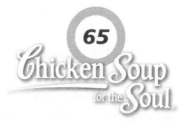

65

The Lion's Prey

The human body can only do so much.
Then the heart and spirit must take over.
~Sohn Kee-chung, 1936 Olympic Marathon Champion

What were you thinking? You can't do this. A marathon! Twenty-six miles is too far. Oh, don't forget the .2. You're too old. You'll die of a heart attack.

There I was, a fifty-year-old grandmother hippo, standing in the middle of young, beautiful, sleek gazelles with taut muscles, ready to bolt at the slightest sound. Jittery gazelles, antelopes, and cheetahs stared at me with wonder in their eyes as if to say, "What are you doing here?" They pranced in place and nervously studied each other as I stood still, wishing I could escape. "BAM!" The cannon blast ripped through the air and bounced off my chest. Instinctively I bolted as if I, too, were a gazelle.

Gazelles, antelope, and cheetahs zipped right, exploded left, and shot past me as they jockeyed for the front, leaving me behind as prey for the lion. Realizing I was not one of those speedy creatures, I slowed to a plodding pace more suitable for a hippo. *You made a mistake. You will never finish. Your mother was right; you will die of a heart attack. That lion, Fear, will surely devour you!*

Sights and sounds blurred. I thought I heard the theme from *Rocky*. I thought I saw cheerleaders waving blue and white pompoms. Mouths seemed to be moving, but all the words melted into a pool of undetectable screams and cheers. It was as if I were in the middle of the jungle with monkeys screeching their warning as the lion approached.

Relax. You can do this. Just enjoy the journey. I took a deep breath for courage and a feeling of tranquility overcame my terror. Instead of trudging like a hippo through the thick sludge of a jungle riverside, I floated like a Snake Eagle across the Serengeti Plain. A smile crept across my face. My breathing united with every gliding step. I started to enjoy the beauty around me. I saw the St. John River as it snaked around newly-built mansions. I saw people waving and yelling. "Good luck number 239." I saw a little girl, bundled in her downy blue parka, standing with her daddy. "Looking good!" A young girl, with long, blond hair blowing gently in the wind, was handing out water. A boy, who could have been a double for Huckleberry Finn, was banging on a pot.

Coach Joe stood on the curbside with his clipboard. *Did he say I'm on pace for Boston? Couldn't be.* Still smiling, I continued to fly across the pavement. I passed one of the beautiful, sleek gazelles. She didn't look very happy. I soared past police officers as they directed traffic around me. I was still floating as I turned right and headed down the last stretch of pavement towards the finish, when WHAM! A vice gripped my legs, squeezing the very life from every muscle like a boa. *But there are only three more miles to go. Oh God, please don't let me fall.* I tried to pick up my feet, but they would only slide as if weighted down by lead. Every move hit my legs with a hammer—a sledgehammer. My brain said, "Go!" My legs said, "No!"

I turned another corner and saw the high school field. I saw the entrance to the track—and the finish line. I kept churning. I heard my name. I started to feel lighter.

The crowd was cheering. I started to glide again. Coach Joe yelled, "You did it! You did it! You're going to Boston!" I sailed around the final curve of the track and through the finish line. All the doubts and fears that were bottled up within me were released, and rose from my toes, propelled through my veins, gathered in my throat, and then gushed from my eyes.

I did do it! Twenty-six point two miles was not too far. I was not too old. I did not die of a heart attack. I beat the lion. I was going to Boston!

~Ginger Herring

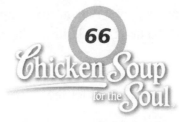

Running for My Life

Prayer may not change things for you, but it for sure changes you for things.
~Samuel M. Shoemaker

I reached my hands out towards the ceiling. "God, please give me a diagnosis, just a diagnosis. That can't be too hard for a great and wonderful God like you." I was desperate. I had been dealing with health issues for years, but the last four years had been spent chained to a crutch and leg brace or imprisoned in a wheelchair.

The initial diagnosis was MS but soon changed to "MS-like symptoms." Thankfully all the neurological tests had come back negative but no one could discover why I lurched around with a gait that Frankenstein's monster would envy. I lost so much strength that some days I couldn't even lift a coffee cup. Now, I had sunk so low that I was trying to coerce God into giving me a diagnosis. I felt utterly hopeless not knowing what was making me so ill.

That dark, silent night, the most wondrous thing happened. As I lay there crying I heard a voice that filled my bedroom. "You're praying for the wrong thing." With that pronouncement came the understanding I longed for.

I sank deeply into the bed, the weight of the world floating off my shoulders and fluttering away.

"God, give me the strength, courage and tools to deal with my life exactly the way it is. Change me, not my situation."

Over the years, I had become my illness. That changed in that single moment. I began to focus on my abilities, whatever they might be, rather than on my limitations. Desperation was no longer my continual companion.

That was the first miracle. The second came six months later when I received the diagnosis that once seemed so crucial for my survival. I learned that I suffered from a rare vitamin deficiency that was causing the main symptoms of my illness.

I immediately threw away the brace. I was confident that I wouldn't need it in the near future. I used the crutch alone for another month until I gained back some strength, but I walked every day. I was determined to use my body as the vitamins started to flow into it and gave it renewed strength.

The first day I timidly trudged around the block with my cane. I wasn't sure I was going to make it as my legs shook and wobbled horribly. However, the second day I traveled two blocks. When I reached a kilometer, I threw away the cane. Soon I could march two and three times that distance.

You couldn't wipe the smile from my face when I was walking. Who knew that the simple action of putting one foot in front of another could inspire such crazy joy? My face hurt from smiling so widely!

It wasn't long before I knew that walking wasn't going to be enough for me. I wanted to run—just because I could! So, I started on the treadmill, praying that my newly able body wouldn't let me down. It didn't.

I ran the first mile almost as slowly as most people walk it, but I ran a whole mile on the first day. I felt as though I had just won the Boston Marathon! Soon I was jogging two and then three miles, five or six times a week. One day the thought came to me that I should run in a race. It was less than a year since I'd received the diagnosis that changed my world and I was running regularly. I knew that I could run a 10K, a quarter of a marathon.

It was a rainy June morning when I set off in the crush of people that were excitedly tackling the streets to run and walk in a local race. I held my breath for the first block, fighting back tears. I, the disabled woman, was running with hundreds of other people. Thank you God! It was a phrase that I would repeat often during that morning.

My goal was to run ten kilometers without walking a step, just because I could. I had trained as hard as I was able to and I thought I was ready… until I arrived at the last kilometer. As I was coming around the bend into the stadium, I heard my weary legs telling my mind, "It's okay to walk a bit. Who will know?"

God heard my legs trying to betray me and set to work.

"Chris!" A familiar voice cried.

One of my colleagues was waving excitedly as she snapped a picture of me.

I smiled and waved back to my friend gratefully.

"I'll know!" I told my legs. "I'll know if I walk!"

Somehow, I found the energy to step it up a notch. I could see the finish line. It came closer and even though my legs kept complaining, I overruled them.

As I stepped over the line, tears spilled down my cheeks.

Three attendants hurriedly approached me. "Are you all right?" each of them inquired with concern.

I had no words to tell them how "all right" I was.

One year, almost to the day, from sitting in a wheelchair and using mobility aids, I had run a 10K. Winning the Boston marathon couldn't have felt as good as that did.

I don't feel as alive as when I'm running. I never take it for granted, being mobile, walking and jogging. Every time I achieve a mile I celebrate and feel exactly as I did the very first time I ran one. The awe and gratitude remains in my life daily.

I was lucky. I never felt useless again after the night of my epiphany. I still pray for God to change me, not my situation. He always gives me the tools I need to run the marathon of life and I sprint the whole way! I show my gratitude with each and every step I run and each person that I smile at today. I truly am running for my life.

~Chris Salstrom

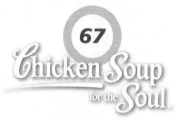

From Smoking to Hot

Do you mind if I don't smoke?
~Groucho Marx

I didn't always run; I smoked instead. I was a smoker for a good nineteen years, if you count when I first started at age eleven, hiding by the train tracks with my friend Mary Alice. Her dad owned the blue-collar town's funeral home. I was hooked early, both physically and mentally, and as I grew older, I loved what smoking did for me. It calmed me down; it revved me up. As a shy adolescent, it gave me something to do with my hands, an activity to fill awkward silences. When I got older, it gave true meaning to the words "cigarette break," back in the days when that was part of the workday. Virginia Slims Menthols were my dear friends, always there, always ready to steady me and give rhythm and structure to my days.

Smokers don't run, and runners usually don't smoke. When I first decided seriously to quit smoking, two months before reaching my thirtieth birthday, I knew I had to replace my three-pack-a-day habit. I could never break any habit unless I replaced it with a new one, and the thought of running to replace smoking seemed a good choice. It would get me out, it would wear me out, and it would be something that I don't associate with smoking, as suggested by several of the self-help books that I had read on the topic. I was always naturally thin, and although this is something I don't really like to admit, I didn't want to gain weight, a side effect of not smoking that my reading had prepared me to accept as inevitable, especially for the first year of being tobacco-free. Running might offset the weight gain, another entry in the plus column.

I was never an athlete. In high school gym I would do a few lame sit-ups before calling it quits. I didn't, and still don't, know the rules of any sport beyond the broad strokes. I didn't own sneakers, or cotton socks, or the then-requisite Walkman. I am optimistic, though, and believe then as now, that I could do whatever I set my mind to. I sprang for the Reeboks, and set out on the road.

I thought running meant, well, running. My first time out, I tore down the road like a gazelle on Starbucks, extra-bold. Within minutes, my lungs burned and the sharp pain in my side slowed me down to a fast walk. I noticed then, a few hundred yards in front of me, another runner, a man who looked like he knew what he was doing. I seemed to be keeping pace with him, even at a walk. Running, I then realized, didn't necessarily mean full-out free running, the seven-year-old kind. Running for exercise was a different kind of thing. I copied the man ahead of me, lifted my knees without increasing my pace, and realized that this is what I should have been doing all along. This felt doable, and so much kinder.

My muscles burned the next morning, but because I have an addictive personality, I kept going. I would try this for a few weeks before I allowed myself to quit, and only then would I make up my mind to continue or not.

That was twenty years ago. I still run, and after that last cigarette on August 15, 1990, I have never smoked another. I run for all the reasons I used to smoke. It relaxes me, it perks me up, and it gives me time and space to think. It keeps me on the slender side, and I believe that it keeps me young in body and mind. I have had to stop for a few weeks to a few months at a time for minor injuries, and once because of a complicated pregnancy. I always miss running, and I always come back.

I run four to six and a half miles at a time, at least four times a week, even with the demands of a challenging job, a family, a full life. I run when I want to remember things, I run to forget, I run as a form of mediation and I run to find solutions to problems, which always seem less complicated and manageable when I am moving.

With only a pair of running shoes, and an old T-shirt as gear, over the years I have conquered my demons and overcome problems that Virginia Slims may not have been up for. Just me, my brain, and my two feet. In rain, in heat, and in sub-freezing weather, I run. I have come a long way, baby.

~*Erika Tremper*

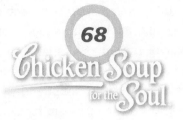

Inspired to Run

Arriving at one goal is the starting point to another.
~John Dewey

I never thought I'd be a "runner."

I was the girl who finished her laps last in gym class. The girl who got winded after two flights of stairs. The girl who complained of blisters after a two-minute jog.

Pretty pathetic, really.

But a few years ago, I changed my tune. I was walking with a group of friends in the Race for the Cure, a 5K race designed to raise money for the fight against breast cancer, when one lady caught my eye.

She was one of the frailest looking women I've ever seen. She must have been close to seventy years old, wearing a bandanna to cover her bald head and a T-shirt with the word "Survivor." She was so small that it seemed as if a swift breeze could tip her over.

But, she was running.

And she was passing me and my group of twenty-something friends.

I couldn't stop staring at her. She ran slowly, but determinedly — as if each step pushed her cancer further into her past. She was practically stomping on her cancer every time her feet touched the ground.

Then, I looked at my friends. Here we were, in the prime of our lives, and this seventy-year-old cancer survivor was kicking our butts!

Right at that moment, I swore that in the next Race for the Cure, I'd be running along with her.

A week later, I found myself at the gym, tentatively approaching the treadmill. I got on and started to jog.

Three minutes after I started, my face was bright red. I was oozing sweat and felt like my lungs were going to burst. I had to slow down to a walk. I thought about the woman at the race. She made it look so easy.

I kept it up.

I was able to go a little longer each time. Three and a half minutes. Four minutes. Five.

A year later, I was at the Race for the Cure again, but this time, I queued with the runners.

When the race started, streams of runners passed me by. But I concentrated on putting one foot in front of the other. One step at a time, I ran forward.

By the second mile, my legs felt like rubber. But I kept moving forward.

As the end of the race approached, I wondered if I'd be able to do it. But then, I remembered the woman from the year before. One foot in front of the other, I ran as fast as I could until I finally crossed that finish line.

The sense of euphoria was incredible. I had just finished my first race! I had run just over three miles without stopping.

I looked down at my legs, amazed. They had done something I'd never thought possible. I have never felt stronger than in that moment.

And, I knew that I wanted to do it again.

~Jennifer Lee Johnson

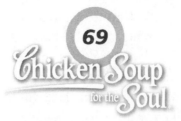

The Most Dedicated

The difference between perseverance and obstinacy is that one comes from a strong will, and the other from a strong won't.
~Henry Ward Beecher

Shortly after graduating from the University of Wisconsin-Whitewater, I secured my first teaching job at Oak Creek High School at the age of twenty-two. In addition to teaching mathematics, my athletic director made me the head varsity women's cross country coach. Being a competitive runner, cyclist, and swimmer since the age of nine, I was very excited about the opportunity to lead a varsity program at the Division I level. Given my high school accomplishments of being an all conference athlete in both cross country and track as well as many great half marathon finishes post high school, I felt that I was properly prepared to get this program on the winning track.

On the first day of practice, I had only twelve girls show up, which is an extremely small number for a big school division team. Most of the girls claimed that they did no running over the summer and consequently we had to start very slow. To make a long story short, it was a very frustrating season for me. Injuries plagued us as many of the girls had hip and knee problems throughout the year, mostly due to their lack of running over the summer months. At the end of the year, we had placed close to the bottom in almost all of the meets. Needless to say I learned quite a bit about coaching and motivating athletes.

After the season had ended, the athletic director informed me that I needed to choose a most valuable runner and a most dedicated runner to award a plaque to at the end-of-year banquet. When it came to choosing the most valuable runner, the decision was easy. A sophomore girl named Bridgette that year improved her time, from last year, by more than 4 minutes in the 2.4 mile cross country race. Besides that, Bridgette was also our number one runner at nearly all of the meets and definitely pushed the other girls on the team during workouts that year.

The decision as to who got the most dedicated runner award was not so easy. I lost several hours of sleep each night trying to figure out who deserved the award. It was not until I looked up the word "dedicated" in the dictionary that it became clear to me.

There was a senior on the team named Andrea who had run on the team all four years. Andrea was by far the slowest runner on the team. She had lots of barriers that made running difficult for her such as asthma, being slightly overweight, and a wobbly running gait. Despite those barriers, Andrea showed more heart, determination, and will in the sport of cross country than I had ever seen from a high school athlete. Her attendance was nearly perfect and she was at all practices on time, which is something that none of the other team members could claim.

When I drove by the high school on off days, I saw Andrea running on the sidewalks getting in extra workouts. During races, she almost always came in dead last, sometimes lagging by more than a quarter of a mile. She always came across the finish line with a smile on her face. The amazing thing is that finishing last did not faze Andrea one bit as she continued to push herself and give it her best. Often times I would run workouts with Andrea as none of the other team members ran at her pace and many times I even offered to make her workout a little shorter and she always declined.

At the final team banquet, I had the honor of awarding Andrea with the most dedicated award. I will never forget how her eyes lit up with amazement and her big smile as she rushed to the podium to claim her plaque. To this day, it was one of the most rewarding moments in my life. After the banquet, many of the parents and athletes questioned my decision, claiming that it should have gone to another girl on the team. The sad truth is that if most of those girls would have had a quarter of the desire that Andrea had, they would have been state athletes.

The next morning I was in my classroom getting ready to teach when Andrea walked in. She looked up at me with tears rolling down her cheeks and said the following words that I will never forget: "That's the first time in my life anyone has ever recognized me for something that I have accomplished and I would just like to thank you." As a tear rolled down my cheek, I looked back at her and told her never to lose her desire and passion for running. Even though my career at Oak Creek High School was short, I have the team picture from that year hung on my apartment wall. Looking at that picture and seeing Andrea in the background sometimes just gives me the inspiration to always do my absolute best in everything that I do.

~Ben Mueller

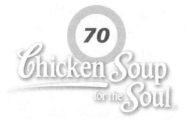

70

The Shelf Curse

Be different, stand out, and work your butt off.
~Reba McEntire

My mother often attributed her robust figure to her German heritage. "In the old country, if the mule was sick, my ancestors strapped the plow to their own backs to work the field," Mom explained while reaching for her fourth slice of cake. "You just wait. The 'shelf curse' will catch up to you one of these days," she warned me.

The "shelf" was a nickname for the derrières grown by the women on my mother's side of the family. Their rears were bountiful to the point of providing a bookshelf-like protrusion under their backs. Growing up I lived in fear, wondering when I would sprout my shelf.

My parents' generation wasn't much on physical activity. They loved to sing, play guitar, tell funny stories and eat. But breaking a sweat wasn't something they did on a regular basis. Running became my way of proving that the cycle of sedentary ways could be broken. I rarely missed a day and kept adding miles. Finally, I set the goal to run a marathon. That would surely break the "shelf curse." I trained religiously until my knees screamed in pain from the impact of pounding the pavement.

"Try using a cushioned track," a runner friend recommended.

That sounded boring, but there was no way I could continue to run on asphalt. Obsessed with breaking the family curse, I took my workout to the track.

It was love at first run. No longer did I have to worry about being hit by a car, tripping over bumps in the sidewalk or dodging dog walkers. I was free to run, run, run, without a care in the world. Soon, I took over the track, and put everything I could ever want on the bench at the quarter-mile mark. I'd drink every two miles, down chocolate energy gel every five miles and change my CD every six miles. I loved getting exact times per loop, and was amazed at how accurately I could pace my tempo. When I really wanted to shake things up, I'd turn around and run in the other direction!

Life with my track was pure bliss. I could practically taste the day I would officially break the family curse, opening the door for my son and daughter to participate in organized sports of their choosing.

I'd reached 14-mile distance runs when disaster struck. In the final two months of my marathon training, school started! Swarms of teenagers, all dressed alike in kelly-green gym clothes, descended on my track. One P.E. class after another, my space had been invaded by the Countryside Middle School Screaming Eagles.

And what strange life forms they were. They hugged the inside lane in clusters, whispering and giggling as I'd run past. They made me self-conscious and I felt like saying, "until you can run as far as me, you'd better keep your mouths shut!" But I didn't want trouble with the teacher. He had the power to banish me and at this point, I was too attached to my track to even consider training elsewhere. Whenever I'd run by his post, I'd lower my gaze and pretend I was oblivious to the fact I was running among thirty adolescents. I even considered wearing green in an attempt to blend.

Then one morning my presence was made obvious when a very astute boy shouted, "Hey, Mr. Lewis… that mom is running on our track again."

Without thinking, I looked up and broke my no-eye-contact rule. Now I had to say something… I jogged up to Mr. Lewis, "I'm not in the way, am I?" I asked as if I'd never noticed the gym class around me.

Before he had time to answer, I blurted out, "I'm training for a marathon, and this is the best surface to run on, my knees were bothering me, it's my first one and it's important that I finish it, there's this family curse I have to break, and…." I held my breath, waiting to be sent to the principal's office.

Mr. Lewis laughed. "Go ahead, keep running. You're good inspiration for the kids. Just keep to the outside."

Ancestors, did you hear that? Someone referred to me as athletic inspiration.

I did complete that marathon!

~Sherrie Page Najarian

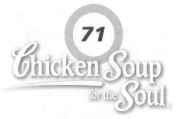

71

First Step

Commit to be fit.
~Author Unknown

I never thought I could be the kind of girl who woke up at 5:20 to run, but here I am doing it. It is still dark outside, my mother and brother are still fast asleep, but I'm putting on my sneakers.

It takes me approximately 10 minutes to brush my teeth, my hair, put my contacts in. iPod in hand, I slowly creep down the hall and peek my head into my mother's room.

"Going to run, Mom," I whisper. "Okay," she sleepily replies.

I happily race down the stairs and open the door to my basement—even after all these years, we still call it the "playroom." That's where my treadmill is.

My treadmill. The place where I can just run and run and be totally relaxed. A year ago, it seemed like a laughable concept that I could run and be relaxed. But now, I like to think of it as my therapy. If I'm angry, I just get on the treadmill and put the speed up as high as I can and just run until I run out all of my anger. I can't be mad after a great workout like that.

You could say my whole obsession with running began because of anger—I was mad at my brother, and, for some reason, I just got on the dormant treadmill my mother was trying to get rid of and started to walk briskly. I could feel the anger—I don't even remember what the fight was about—starting to boil over. In a sudden burst of energy, I turned the treadmill up to five miles an hour.

I laugh at that now—five miles an hour, a 12-minute mile,

seems like such an easy jog to me now. But back then I was huffing and puffing after 2 minutes. I was about to turn it down again when the mile time flashed on the screen—12 minutes. I could do 12 minutes, couldn't I?

I could, but I was so tired after that I felt like I never wanted to move again. Yet, I felt at the same time… empowered. Like nothing could hold me back. So, a little while later I ran another mile. And another. By the end of that day, I had run three miles—an amazing feat for an out-of-shape, overweight girl like me.

I never let go of running. I began a system—run a mile, walk a mile, rest. Later, run another mile, walk another mile. I averaged four miles a day. A definite improvement from my normal exercise of lazily walking my dogs half a mile.

That treadmill, which my mother once wanted to get rid of, became the place where I spent hours a day. Soon, I was running two miles straight before doing any walking. Then, I cut out walking all together—I was just running. I could run for up to an hour and a half, no stopping. My old jeans began to feel loose on me. I was elated. I hadn't gotten into this to lose weight, but this was a happy side effect.

Running then led to a gym membership. The equipment there was amazing—rows and rows of treadmills, exercise bikes, a huge room full of every single kind of weight machine one could imagine…. I was in heaven.

One of the reasons I believe I have been so successful in fitness is I am not afraid to push myself. Run an extra mile? No problem. Five miles an hour? Please, I can do it at 6.5. An extra hundred crunches, ten more pounds, one more set of lunges, it was all so much fun. I truly enjoyed fitness…. I do still truly enjoy fitness.

Now, I go to the gym six days a week. I do not have to force myself to go—it is something I really love to do.

Of course, my favorite thing to do is run—which is why I run three miles every day at the gym and wake myself up half an hour early each morning so I can run two miles before school.

I never joined a track team, or entered any races. My only

competition is myself. I went from being a lazy, overweight girl who barely moved herself from in front of the TV to someone who is truly fit, with muscles and a small waist. I've gone down to a size 4, but even those pants are loose on me. But weight isn't really what it's all about—it's the wonderful way I see myself now. The accomplished feeling I get every day.

Trust me, if I can get into shape, anyone can. It doesn't matter your age—I began when I was thirteen. All you have to do is take that first step.

~Fallon Kane

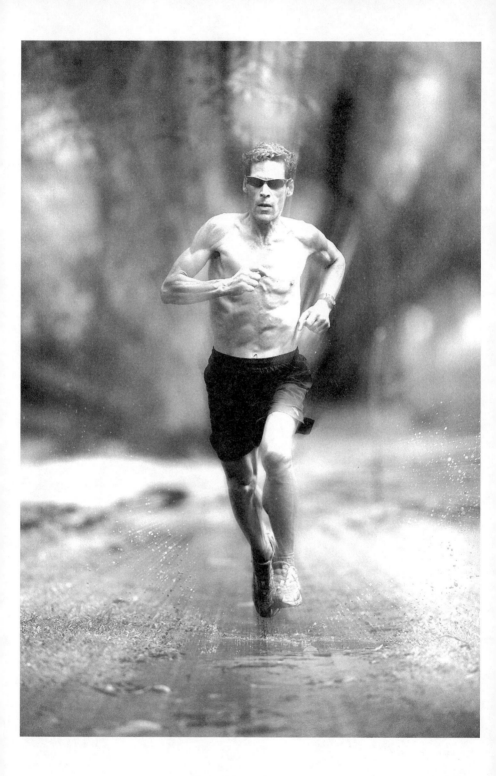

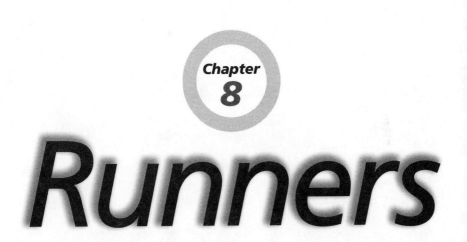

Chapter
8

Runners

Fortitude

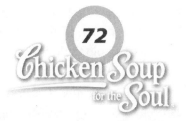

72

Listen to Yourself

It is not the mountain we conquer but ourselves.
~Edmund Hillary

In April 2003, we adopted our daughter, Annabella. This occurred in the same year I set my most challenging athletic goal — completing the Grand Slam of ultrarunning and the Badwater 135 in the same year.

The Grand Slam consists of four of the hardest 100-mile trail races in the USA: Western States 100 in Squaw Valley, California (June), the Vermont 100 in Woodstock (July), the Leadville 100 in Colorado (August), and the Wasatch 100 in Utah (September).

The Badwater 135 is the hardest, hottest foot race on Earth (it is not uncommon for the soles of one's shoes to melt). It's a 135-mile run from the lowest point in the continental U.S., (282 feet below sea level) to the portals of Mt. Whitney, at an elevation of 8,300 feet.

The first thing people said to me when Annabella arrived was, "I guess you won't be able to compete in the races you wanted to this season." I heard this repeatedly and even once from my husband Jay. He thought I might have to "narrow it down." I thought about this for about one second and said, "I must try; I have set this goal, I'll raise thousands of dollars for needy children, and I will be the only male or female to ever accomplish this." I did not want to turn back.

Parents know all about sleep deprivation and the loss of time for yourself. I didn't want to sleep because all I wanted to do was look at Annabella. Thus, my training was cut by more than fifty percent. So I made a new goal: "Do the best you can with the time you have and don't worry about it. One race at a time, one step at a time, one breath at a time." I felt certain of myself despite the fact that people continued to say, "She won't be able to do it."

At the Western States 100, Annabella did not sleep well the night before the race so I was beat going into it. I don't remember much of those last 30 miles because I was sleep-walking and running. As I crossed the finish line, there was Annabella asleep in her stroller. I looked up and gave thanks.

For the Vermont 100 Annabella and Jay stayed home. It was very difficult to spend time away from my family but I finished the race in style, slept for three hours, boarded a plane and set out to run the Badwater 135.

I had run the Badwater 135 five times, but this time was the hardest. At 100 miles I felt I could not go on any longer. I was in excruciating pain. I was going to throw in the towel. Then I got word from one of my crew members that Jay and Annabella were driving all the way to the finish line (a 20-hour drive) to meet me. So I slept for a few hours, they arrived and I got my butt up and finished the race. I was more determined than ever before in my life. I was running strong and I was on fire!

The entire Leadville 100 race takes place at over 10,500 feet. I was doing great until the last 15 miles. I was so tired from running all night that I couldn't envision finishing. One of my good friends and my husband were on my crew and knew that the one thing that sets me on fire is getting me mad. So they did. I took off — passing about 75 other people.

The Wasatch 100 is hard. The last 10 miles will eat you up if you have run the first 90 miles too hard. It thundered and stormed through part of the night but I continued to race. This was the last race — all I had to do was get to the finish line. One step at a time, one mile at a time. With seven miles left Jay told me I was in second place for the women. This was shocking to me. I hadn't worried about how I would place — I only focused on getting to the finish line. Normally I would have tried to keep second place but God told me over and over again, "It does not matter what place you are in;

what matters is that you're about to accomplish your goal and raise thousands of dollars for children."

I ran the last mile hard and cried and lifted my hands up giving thanks—I did it! We did it! You see, this was never just about me running all those miles. It was about my family and the love, support and belief that they instilled in me. It was about trusting what God was telling me, not what everyone else had to say. At the awards ceremony I was given the first place award for all the women who had set out to run the Grand Slam. I looked at my husband, my daughter and the friends who had helped me get this award and said, "We did it!"

Never let anyone tell you that you can't do something. If you fail, you still win by trying. Surround yourself with people who will support you and believe in you. Most of all believe in yourself and give thanks. Always give thanks. I went to sleep that night after the last race with Annabella sleeping on my stomach and Jay next to me. That was my greatest reward. If I can do it, you can do it. One step at a time.

~Lisa Smith-Batchen

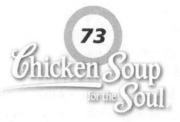

73

My Love for Ultrarunning

Do or do not. There is no "try."
~Jedi Master Yoda

I was only three years old when my dad (Doug Malewicki) took me on my first overnight backpacking trip to San Gorgonio Mountain. I can still remember hiking up the Vivian Creek Trail carrying my bright orange backpack filled with a jacket and a stuffed animal. One trip, that's all it took for the mountains to get in my blood.

Every summer, my dad and I took weeklong backpacking trips to Tuolumne Meadows in Yosemite National Park. I loved every aspect of hiking different trails and living outside in nature.

Fast forward three decades later. I continued the tradition that my dad began. It was August 2002 and my daughter Sierra, who I named after my favorite mountain range, was two and a half years old. My dad and I took Sierra on her first backpacking trip to the Minarets in Mammoth, California. Every summer since, Sierra, my dad and I have gone on hiking trips together. We have hiked the John Muir Trail and all over Tuolumne Meadows. It is one of my dreams to run the 211-mile John Muir trail.

I was drawn to trail running after my daughter Sierra was born a decade ago. My dad bought me a jogging stroller. I used it every day until the tires were completely bald. My dad encouraged me to sign up for a Winter Trail Running Series. The WTRS consists of trail races every other Saturday in the Cleveland National Forest. The race series starts with a 12K in January and culminates with the 50K in

March. The San Juan Trail 50K was my first ultra in March of 2003. I was immediately hooked on the ultramarathon distance.

In December 2004, I had a minor setback when I broke my left ankle (fibula) on a 22-mile training run. After being in a hard cast and crutches for two months I was ready to get back to running and training. I became friends with Dean Karnazes that year. Dean's book *Ultramarathon Man: Confessions of an All-Night Runner* inspired me like nothing else. I wanted to get faster, train harder and do my best at races. I started incorporating mountain biking and swimming into my training regime. Crosstraining is my secret weapon for helping me recover from racing and winning ultras on back to back weekends for over a month straight.

From 2000 until 2010, I have accumulated forty ultramarathon wins and more than a dozen trail marathon wins and even a handful of half-marathon and 10K wins. I won more ultramarathons than any man or woman in 2007. I broke five course records over a six-week time period. My course record streak in 2007 consisted of four 50Ks and one 50-miler. The one week in between that I did not race, I ran 75 miles over Memorial Day weekend with Gordy Ainsleigh, the founder of the Western States 100-Mile Endurance Run. The Western States trail is one of my most favorite trails in the world. It is so beautiful. Thanks to Gordy Ainsleigh, who was the first person to ever run the Western States 100-mile race in 1974, we are able to experience running 100 miles from Squaw Valley to Auburn on the Western States trail. The amazing Winged God, Gordy is one of my best friends. I paced him at the Western States 100 in 2006 and 2007 and plan to do so again in 2010.

My dad got me interested in trail running and in return I got my dad interested in running ultramarathons. My dad has run many 50K races. My dad even ran 70 miles to celebrate his 70th birthday. His motto for the three-day event was that famous quote from Jedi Master Yoda in *Star Wars*, "Do or do not. There is no 'try.'"

On January 23, 2010, three generations of my family toed the line at the Winter Trail Running Series 15K race. Sierra, age ten, finished the 9.2-mile trail race with over 3,500 feet of vertical ascent in

1:54. She won first place for all male and female competitors under age nineteen. She even beat her grandpa by 12 minutes.

I can picture our ancestors looking down on us and wondering why modern day humans would choose to run 30, 50, 100 or more miles just for the pleasure and pure challenge. I am grateful to use my mind and body to run trails and feel free like a wild horse roaming, racing and exploring beautiful trails with forests, meadows, peaks and valleys.

You are a rich person if you experience trail running. Different trails have different personas. Some are nasty and rocky and steep. Some are sweet and smooth as sugar. Races can keep things exciting and new. There are so many trails to explore and so many new races to run to keep the sport exciting.

Ultrarunning makes you truly live in the moment, one step at a time. It takes you down to the basics. Drink, eat and perpetual forward motion. You experience the highest highs, the lowest lows and everything in between. The people, the pain, the challenge, the struggle and the achievement makes it all worth it.

The bond that develops between runners is unmatched in most human endeavors. In the longer events we sometimes suffer together. I truly consider my ultra friends part of my family.

My best trail running moment was a few years ago when I won the Javelina Jundred 100-mile race in 19 hours and 42 minutes. Everything clicked and it was magic! In 2006 and 2007 I won the Orange Curtain 100K, the Twin Peaks 50K, and the Orange Curtain 50K and I beat ALL the GUYS at all three events! That was AWESOME!! The ultrarunning guys don't seem to mind getting "chicked" by me.

The greatest advice I have to give to someone who wants to start running ultras is to never stop believing in yourself. Remain tough, stay strong, and prove the naysayers wrong. Since I started running ultramarathons in 2003, I am more confident that I have ever been. I can run 100 miles in under twenty hours, and therefore I feel that I am capable of doing anything that I set my mind to, if I want it bad enough.

~Michelle Barton

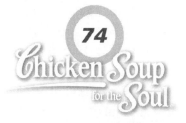

74

40 on 40

Just remember, once you're over the hill you begin to pick up speed.
~Charles Schultz

4 0 on 40... That pretty much says it all. Rather than black balloons and the usual morbid celebratory rituals, I chose a different way to celebrate. I decided to celebrate my 40th birthday running my body into the ground. That's right, 40 miles on my 40th birthday!

I have run every day of my life for the last ten years. Running strengthens me in many ways... physically, emotionally and spiritually. The world is absolutely perfect during my run... rain, sleet or snow.

It was 2:00 AM and I was lying in bed waiting to start my 40 miles, I had a crew of friends and supporters ready to run with me at various legs of the course, starting bright and early at 5:00 AM!

At 2:45 AM I got up and dressed and e-mailed everyone to say "I am heading out!" I began my run. The first six miles in the dark, not a sound. It was a clear summer morning in Iowa. A bit humid, but comfortable and peaceful and motivating knowing that I was the only creature out moving this time of the day. After about four miles and about 3:30 in the morning, a friend and fellow biker came upon me to check and make sure I was doing okay. An hour later, I returned home for a drink of water and headed back out the door. You see, I was running a 6.5 mile loop six times and a one miler at the end. This running ritual continued with various friends and community supporters running with me, riding their bikes alongside, or driving by and honking and yelling "Happy Birthday!"

I live in a small town of about 15,000 people. The local newspaper decided to cover the story of my 40-mile run. It made the front page. I thought that was really neat, but what if I didn't make it? Yikes! So, I got out there and ran.

Several hours and miles later, the day turned hot and humid. It was a typical Iowa July day. My friends and pacers kept me entertained as I put one foot in front of the other. I'd run several marathons and made it through the first 26.2 miles. There were only 14.8 miles to go! So, I kept running. I had people along the route who had coolers on their lawns loaded with water and Diet Mountain Dew (the true beverage of choice for distance runners, or at least for me). Bathrooms were plentiful on the run, although not needed due to the heat and dehydration.

My pace was slowing, but my crew was encouraging. Mile 35. Counting down. One foot in front of the other, feet aching, arms heavy by my side. I was wondering why I was doing this. Then mile 40! I was home with my crew. I began to cry, from relief that it was over, that I ran 40 miles without killing myself, and most importantly, that my friends took time from their busy day to spend a few hours supporting my mission, because they were friends. Now that is friendship and that is running to me. I realized at that moment that I was surrounded by a small community of people who loved and cared for me.

We wrapped up the day with a great big bash at our local country club. On Cloud 9 and feeling great. I went home, and thought about the wonderful day. Got up the next morning and went about my day as always, ready for the next endeavor. I remember telling everyone that was the best birthday of my life!

And then… several days later it was brought to my attention that I was one of the top "blogged" people in Newton that week. I questioned why I was being blogged in the local paper. So, being human, I had to go online and check it out. Many blogs were supportive and encouraging. But just one or two negative comments can rip your heart out.

This is what was written: "Who does she think she is, Paris Hilton? Running around the town in practically nothing! She's insane!" and… "Isn't there anything else going on in town that's more important? This is ridiculous news."

With the numerous positive comments and supporters, just two negative blogs brought me down… but not for long. You see, a lesson was learned from this experience.

I learned that not only could my body endure 40 long miles completed in 7.5 hours, but my mind could endure the 40 miles. I realized that life is about what you think and what you say to yourself when you are alone.

~Melissa Butler

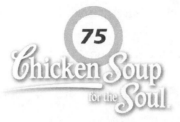

75

A Lesson in Running

We may train or peak for a certain race, but running is a lifetime sport.
~Alberto Salazar

It was my first marathon. Philadelphia, November, 6 AM. The wind and the rain chilled me to the bone and the sun wasn't yet out to warm up the air. The corral was full. Packed with runners standing arm to arm, jogging in place to stay warm. The starting horn would go off any second. You could feel the tension in the air. I was ready. I was twenty-eight and in the best shape of my life.

At least, I thought I was. Sure, I was fit. Even though I had only been running for a few months, I ran all the time and had run several races already. But none of them were 26.2 miles. The farthest I had run before was only fifteen miles. Still, I was young and cocky and I knew I could do it.

The horn went off and the race started. The crowd surged forward. A mob of running sneakers. It was exciting. The adrenaline kicked in and the weather became the furthest thing from my mind. I just concentrated on the cheers of the crowd and holding my own position amongst the other runners. I had no real finishing goal in mind, but when the crowd dispersed and I was settled into my pace I soon calculated that I could easily break four hours.

A few miles in I ran past an elderly runner. He must have been seventy years old and I was surprised he was even in the race. I was even more surprised that he was still ahead of me. He kept to the side of the road, his old legs moving one in front of the other, slowly but methodically. I passed him up without giving him a second glance or a word of encouragement.

As the miles wore on people were dropping out left and right but I kept moving. Fifteen miles came and went and I was on pace to beat four hours. Then, something strange happened.

I started to get tired. Very tired. It happened all at once. One second my stride was feeling fine, and then the next each step became harder and harder. My goal of four hours soon got pushed back to 4:10. Then 4:20. Finally, at about the 20-mile mark, I couldn't run anymore. I had to walk.

I moved to the side of the road and plodded along. I needed a second wind, but it wasn't coming. The rain was back. A cold rain soaking into my clothes and my sneakers. Now, people were passing me. I had hit the dreaded wall and there was nothing I could do about it but concentrate on putting one foot in front of the other.

Then, the elderly man passed me. He looked the same as he had earlier. Running at the same speed. As he passed, he looked over at me and smiled.

"Only a few more miles to go, lad. Don't stop now!"

The thought of being beaten by a seventy-year-old man got me moving again. Like I said, I was young and cocky, and this little setback had only dampened my confidence a little. If I got moving I would be able to beat 4:30 and pass up that old man again.

So I moved up from a shambling walk to a shambling jog. The elderly gentleman had run ahead of me but I could still see him in the distance, moving forward at that same pace.

I spent the rest of the race trying to catch him, but no matter how hard I tried I wasn't getting any closer. The finish line grew nearer, the crowds on the sidewalks got bigger and louder and that helped me to run faster and faster. Soon, I was running at a good pace with my second wind but the elderly man still stayed just out of reach. He didn't stop at all. He just kept running and running.

He crossed the finish line ahead of me and I was soon to follow at 4:28:45. I never had such mixed emotions. I was proud and elated at finishing the marathon, but I was angry with myself for letting that elderly gentleman beat me. In the finishers' tent, after grabbing a handful of bananas and some water, I tried to find him but he was gone.

It was only later on that I realized how much I admired him.

I'll never forget that man. The senior citizen runner who put the cocky twenty-eight-year-old in his place. Some day I hope to be like him, running marathons in my seventies and passing all those first-timers as they struggle to finish. I'll make sure to give them encouragement.

"Only a few more miles to go! Don't stop now, lad!"

I know the real encouragement won't come from my words, but it will come later when they look back on that race. When they realize that they have only just started their running careers. That the real test of a runner is not running for just 26.2 miles.

It is running for a lifetime.

~P.R. O'Leary

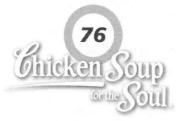

76

Changing My Story

Relish the bad training runs. Without them it's difficult to recognize, much less appreciate, the good ones.
~Pat Teske

The marathon appeared on my cosmic to-do list in only my second year of running. The 26.2-mile run seemed like the perfect challenge to demonstrate to the world—and myself—my transformation from perennial fat girl to healthy runner. Not only would I complete the marathon, I thought, but I would run it in my conservative, but still respectable, goal time.

But just a few weeks before the race, my marathon dreams crashed down around me after the worst run of my life.

The afghan blanket was pulled up to my chin. My legs were elevated with extra pillows at the end of the couch and my ankles and knees were packed in ice. I couldn't stop the tears. The goal had been to run for 3 hours and 15 minutes—my final long run before beginning to taper for the marathon. I had pace goals and intentions of completing the workout perfectly so that mentally I would be confident and focused for the biggest physical challenge of my life.

Only, I completely broke down.

My knees started hurting. My pace slowed. I started crying during the run. A flood of negative thoughts that started as whispers turned into forceful shouts. Who was I to start running at age thirty-four? Who was I to run a marathon? Who was I to call myself an athlete?

The 3 hours and 15 minutes ticked off painfully and slowly. I slogged through the cold May morning in western New York State, wondering if I even had the right to call what I was doing "running."

I had always believed the innate qualities needed to be an athlete were missing from my genetic code. I had started running to challenge myself, to see what might happen if I tried. While huddled on the couch packed in ice after breaking down on what was supposed to be my marathon "test run," feelings of failure swept over me.

A few days later, my friends were trying to cheer me up, relating tales of their own training breakdowns and catastrophic races. I had met all these people through running. A run with one led to meeting another and another and another. Eventually, I found that I had created a new tribe for myself—one that was positive and encouraging. A tribe of people who believed in me even when I doubted myself.

Feeling a sense of security, I shared with them my "fat pictures"—photos from my college years when I was fifty pounds heavier. Weight was always an issue for me and the buffet line at the dining hall coupled with late night pizza and beer meant I easily packed on the pounds.

"Look how fat I was," I pointed out.

"But still pretty," my friend, Sue, said. Funny. That never occurred to me. I was fat. How could I be pretty? Even now, my figure flaws were plenty. There were numerous areas where the loss of a few pounds would make me look better and might even make me a faster runner.

Sue's comment triggered an idea. During the marathon, along with my gels, I would carry one of those fat photos. At some point on the course, I would ball it up and throw it away. I would forget about the fat pictures.

The marathon wall hit me around Mile 16. What started as a cloudy May morning with drizzle turned into a humid, sun-blazing affair. And by the time I got to Mile 22, I was near tears. My pace was all wrong, just like that horrible, horrible run a few weeks earlier. I was in pain. I was walking. I was terribly upset with myself.

Reaching into my pocket to take another gel, my hand brushed against my fat photo. This was the place to dump it. I took it out, looked at it and said goodbye. The photo crumpled easily in my now gooey hand and floated through the air as I tossed it into the garbage can.

What was I saying goodbye to? Oddly enough, I wasn't bidding adieu to my former fat self. Because running had taught me that it was never about the weight. It was only about how I chose to define myself.

I could be a runner anytime I wanted, at any pace I wanted, if only that's what I believed. It didn't matter how fast I was going, or if I was walking, or where I placed in my age group. It didn't matter how fast or slow anybody else ran. The comparison and the final time are just for our amusement—a game to keep us interested. The running, I learned, was about the doing and the being. Being attached to any specific outcome was yet another way to impose a limiting definition on myself. And running was teaching me to be open to possibilities, not closed up with old patterns.

I threw away the old picture, not to rid my existence of my former self but to exorcise the way in which I viewed myself—past and present. I threw away those old definitions. I decided I was an athlete. I decided I was a runner. And I decided that no matter how long it took me to finish my first marathon, no one could denigrate that accomplishment except for me. I threw away the self-doubt and comparisons at that water stop.

I continued for the next 4.2 miles grateful for that horrible training run. Grateful that it broke me, that it made me question who my authentic self really was. As my foot bled from blisters and my muscles burned from the miles, I knew I had been here before. And this time, I knew the way out.

~Amy Moritz

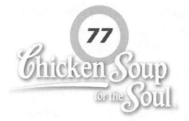

77
Chicken Soup for the Soul

Running with Joy

It's not your finishing time that's important but the kind of time you have finishing.
~Art Castellano, Director New Jersey Marathon

While every marathon is 26.2 miles, New York's is special because of its sold-out field of 38,000 international participants, the thunderous cheers for the runners throughout the five-borough course, and—well—because it's New York City. The 2008 marathon was my second New York City Marathon and my fourteenth marathon overall. While it was my slowest marathon, it nevertheless would be one of my most memorable.

The day before the marathon, I had lunch with eighty-one-year-old Joy Johnson, who was about to run her twenty-first consecutive NYC Marathon—a streak that very few have accomplished. Joy still had the competitive juices flowing through her, as a younger rival, a champion runner the prior year, had entered the eighty to eighty-five age group to challenge her for first place. Joy was determined to better her 2007 winning time. She had stepped up her training regimen, including fifty miles of running each week plus speed work, hill-repeats, and running on stadium steps. Joy had been coached by former Olympian Jeff Galloway and at the Dick Beardsley running camps. Indeed, I first met Joy at Jeff's annual summer camp where we bonded during breakfasts after the morning's wake-up jog. Because we were again enjoying each other's company at our lunch with family and friends, Joy asked me to "pace her," to stay close to her sub-six-hour goal for the marathon. I happily accepted the challenge.

On marathon Sunday, Joy was eager to run; I had to keep reminding her to slow down during the start and stay on the agreed pace. Our strategy was to run for 2 minutes and then to walk a stretch to conserve our legs and reduce the adrenaline rush. We had many bridges to cross before we would cross the finish line in Central Park near the Tavern on the Green. It was important that we conserve our energy. The start was across the two-mile-long Verrazano Bridge. We dashed through Brooklyn for the next eleven miles, followed by a quick hop over the Pulaski Bridge for a short visit to the borough of Queens. At mile 15 we pounded up the ramp of the 100-year-old 59th Street Bridge feeling groovy. We cantered this mile-long stretch leading back into Manhattan, our hearts pounding in anticipation of stepping onto First Avenue, where the largest and loudest bunch of fans waited for the runners and their final ten miles of the marathon. The sound of the cheers in many languages coalesced with the sight of all the colorful running outfits from France, Mexico, Japan, Spain, and other countries. We had huge smiles on our faces and goose-bumps on our arms that had nothing to do with the cold, windy day.

Family and friends lined the avenue. We made time for quick hugs and nourishment of energy gels, concentrated paste that we call "vanilla frosting," washed down by water. As we made our way up the avenue, we knew the fastest runners had long gone by. It was now a people's run and the folks on the sidelines did not disappoint, her admirers shouting "Go Joy," and others cheering "Go CERT Will," the "CERT" a reference to my proudly worn embossed shirt honoring my volunteer colleagues in the Community Emergency Response Team.

Joy was on target for her sub-six-hour time when she got leg cramps after mile 18 that almost caused her to fall. Joy leaned on my arm as she pressed her fingers into the cramp but worried aloud that she was now out of the race. At this moment, my role changed from pacing Joy to helping her regain mental focus. I kept us moving and reached out for help. From another runner who had salt packets, Joy spilled some on the back of her hand and licked the salt to recoup sodium into her blood stream. Then, luckily, we spotted a local coach who always sported the biggest smile, cheering everyone on the course. We were relieved to realize he was holding "the stick" that runners use to massage cramped limbs. We did a quick stick massage on Joy's calf to break down the cramp. To my delight, Joy was receptive to my suggestions to change to a quick, short walking stride with head held high, back of neck elongated, eyes scanning ahead, shoulders relaxed, and arms swinging backwards as if hitting a bar with the elbows. Joy soldiered on and waited for her body to tell her when she could start to run again.

We finally trotted into the Bronx via the Willis Avenue Bridge, a tough spot as mile 20 is called the "runner's wall" that separates those who ran smart from those who were hurting. Since we had run smart, we galloped over the Madison Avenue Bridge back into Manhattan. Looping back into Central Park, we felt a surge of energy knowing we had only two miles to go. We left the park one last time at East 59th Street and, jogging towards Columbus Circle, we could see ourselves on the JumboTron. We did a quick check to be sure we were smear-free—we wanted to look good for our finisher's photo. We did it—and Joy was again first in her age group, shaving over 50 minutes from her 2007 win! When Joy jogged the final two miles, I had the biggest smile of all because I made a difference by being there for her, every step of the way.

With our finishers' medals draped over us, I escorted Joy to her midtown hotel and then I floated home to the East 60s. What kind of time did we have? Priceless!

~William Sanchez

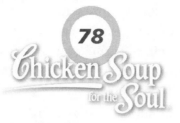

78

Running through Denial

I ran and ran every day, and I acquired a sense of determination, this sense of spirit that I would never, never, give up, no matter what else happened.
~Wilma Rudolph

I ran my very first marathon in New York City in 2005. One week later I went into the hospital for a hysterectomy. What a difference a week makes!

My first question to the oncologist when he told me I needed surgery was "can it wait until after the marathon?" I was more than two-thirds of the way through my sixteen-week training program by then, and I just could not fathom all those miles accrued for nothing. When I look back at that time now, the marathon posed a huge distraction for me, and I desperately needed that. I could not face the diagnosis of cervical cancer, and I preferred to operate in denial. Don't get me wrong… I was diligent about getting all of my tests and routinely following up with my doctor. I just never got my brain around the word "carcinoma" as a synonym for cancer. So while I was awaiting test results and being referred to an oncologist (another scary word to me), I continued to run. My training became an escape. And in that dark time, I received some good news; I could run the marathon and schedule the surgery afterwards.

It is funny how when you are dealing with a crisis, your definition of "good news" can change drastically. Two years earlier, my goal was to avoid a hysterectomy when my doctor first made the diagnosis of carcinoma in situ (the diagnosis that I somehow did not equate to cancer at the time). Luckily, my prayers were answered then, and

I ended up having a less invasive surgery. Good news! But then a routine test came back abnormal in the fall of 2005, and I was faced with no other option. First, of course, I wanted to know if I was going to die. When the oncologist assured me I wouldn't, all of a sudden a hysterectomy did not sound so bad.

I then wanted to know if I could continue my pursuit of the marathon—the race that represented so much to me, especially now that it was in jeopardy of being taken away. At some point during the training, the marathon takes on an importance that goes beyond running twenty to forty miles per week. It became a personal challenge to push my body to a limit that seemed crazy even to me, but somehow prove to myself in the process that I could accomplish this feat and do it despite my health crisis.

The training is brutal. I do not know how people run this race more than once. The first time you do not know what to expect: the toll it takes on your body and the obsession that overtakes your mind. For sixteen weeks, it is all you can think about, talk about and do! For me, this became my salvation. I could focus on running, not cancer, and it did not require any additional mental effort to pull that off. The training was so demanding that it naturally occupied both my brain and body. Even when I slept, I dreamt about running. I wanted to be prepared, and I was strict about following the training program exactly how it was written. I did not want to get injured, and I certainly wanted to finish the race running, not walking. So I ran every long run, and I choked down protein gels, and I read books about marathon training, and I bathed my sore muscles. And through it all, I reminded myself that all my hard work would be rewarded at the finish line.

Looking back now, I realize that I was living in denial. I had "tricked" my brain to block out all thoughts of cancer. I convinced myself that if I did not talk about it, it did not exist, and as a result, many people did not know what I was going through. I preferred it that way, which was very ironic because I am naturally gregarious and open. During this time, however, I became reserved and private. Cancer became sort of a taboo subject. Running dominated most conversations anyway, and it was certainly a more pleasant topic. Again, since it was my first marathon, every aspect of training for this race was interesting, exciting and worth sharing. I wanted to share, but only on my terms.

As brutal as the training was, the actual day of the marathon was magical. There was nothing like the feeling of running through New York City neighborhoods with thousands of spectators cheering and live music blaring. Rounding that turn beyond the Queensboro Bridge onto First Avenue at the 18-mile mark was the closest I have ever come to being a rock star! What a feeling to emerge from the long stretch of the bridge into the sunlight again and to see screaming "fans" packed ten deep on the sidewalk. I took every bit of that energy and harnessed it into my steely resolve to finish the race strong. I ran beside a 6'3" man dressed as Wonder Woman, complete with the wig and cape, for the last five miles. The funny thing about the marathon in New York City is plenty of people run it in outlandish costumes. Wonder Woman was one of the tamer ones—there was one runner dressed up as the Statue of Liberty, juggling throughout the race! Obviously everyone shows up on race day with his or her own agenda. I had mine too.

My finish line photo, with Wonder Woman right behind me, hangs on my wall now. I did it! I used to say that I admired people who ran marathons but that I never could. I proved myself wrong. I knew I could take that same determination into the operating room one week later and apply it to my recovery. And I still had a whole week to wear my medal and bask in the glory of my marathon experience. I learned a lot about myself in 2005. I turned forty, I got cancer, and I ran a marathon. Somehow I survived all three milestones with a little courage (and a lot of denial!) that I discovered along the way.

~Julie Bradford Brand

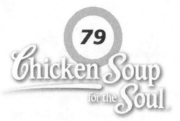

79

When Life Hands You a Lemon

Win or lose you will never regret working hard, making sacrifices, being disciplined or focusing too much. Success is measured by what we have done to prepare for competition.
~John Smith

I grew up listening to Bill Stern, the famous sports announcer. What I remember most is how Bill Stern signed off when he finished broadcasting: "It's not whether you win or lose—it's how you play the game."

Those philosophical words were a great help to me in regard to the 2009 marathon in Newport, Oregon. A fully-official marathon had been on my bucket list since both my daughter and granddaughter ran the LA Marathon. For years they'd been saying to me, "Hey, you can do it, too."

I may be seventy-five years young, but I've spent my whole life keeping fit and setting goals. In my forties, I decided to run six 10Ks, just for the challenge. I discovered what "runner's high" feels like, and I still have those six T-shirts.

I also set a goal to ride my bicycle from the Canadian border to Mexico on Highway 101 before turning fifty. Did that, too, with one gal-pal and no sag wagon. We did not plan on "sagging," and never did.

In February 2009 I took a deep breath and signed up for the Newport Marathon. I invested in top-notch running shoes, an excellent pedometer and carefully kept track of my training miles. I found a group of women (all of whom were twenty years younger than me, but just as determined to conquer their first marathon). These women were into power-walking, as their bodies, like mine, let us know that full-out running was not going to cut it.

Power-walking felt doable and, after all, most folks of any age can put one foot in front of the other and walk. Our group met almost every day to train. We all lost weight and our bodies grew stronger. I loved the camaraderie of these women and our growing excitement about the coming marathon. Until one day the youngest and most athletic gal in our group said, "We better start taking some hills."

Ooops. Big mistake. At least one of the women had trouble breathing and fell behind. My problem was a sudden sharp pain in my right hip. The pain was constant, relentless and eventually forced me to our doctor's office. "Bursitis," he said.

"Bursitis?" I exclaimed. "Isn't that for old people?" We agreed on a cortisone shot. The pain let up and I rejoined my group. When they took to the hills, I continued to train on the flats.

The weeks were flying past and the numbers in my mileage journal were adding up. I felt pumped and ready. "Bring on that marathon," I said to myself, ignoring the pain I felt in my toe. I didn't look and I didn't want to know.

And then—just two days before the marathon, I made myself look at that toe. It was bright red and incredibly painful.

"Why are you limping?" my husband asked. "Is it your bursitis again?" He's eighty-two and I think he enjoyed the thought that his wife was somewhat normal.

"Don't even ask," I said, and went back to the doctor.

"Hmm," said the doctor, examining my bright, red toe and the nail that was turning black. "You have a badly-infected toe. I'm putting you on antibiotics."

"Huh?" I said. "But what about the marathon?"

"Well," he said. "You can still do it, but you'll be limping the entire way—and then your back will go out." I gimped out of his office in tears. I drove home totally depressed.

But then, a couple of things happened: my husband, who is brilliant with numbers, asked to see my "mileage notebook," and within seconds informed me that I had power-walked exactly 453 miles since sending in the entry form and the amount of miles figured out to be roughly seventeen marathons.

It also dawned on me that all that training had made me healthier and in better shape than I'd been in years. About then, Bill Stern's words flashed into my brain and turned the negative feelings of "oh poor me" into "what can I do to be a positive part of the marathon?"

Voilà, I thought. They must need volunteers! Organizations and events always need volunteers.

I picked up the phone, started networking with various people and ended up with the perfect volunteer job—for me and my aching black toe. Riding in one of the vans going back and forth along the marathon route, playing cheerleader to those on the road who seemed to be floundering.

You could feel and see them perk up when those of us in the van hollered out encouragement. I forgot my own disappointment as I saw all those runners, walkers, including my own power-walking group, and several wheelchair contenders.

And there were, as happens in most major sports events, the few who could no longer go on and needed to be picked up and taken for some medical help. I also thought of the people who train four years for the Olympics and then do not make the team.

I will never forget the young Asian girl who came here from San Francisco for this marathon. Her second attempt. We found her curled up on the side of the road, in a fetal position. It was mile 22 and she had developed horrible leg cramps. We picked her up and I scooched over in the back seat of the van so she could stretch out, her head in my lap, crying from pain and frustration. I held her and told her I could understand her disappointment, that there would be other marathons and to "never ever give up on your dreams."

This is a perfect example of what to do when life hands you a lemon—make lemonade. And if you ever know someone who has set a big goal only to not make it—remind them of Bill Stern's words:

"It's not whether you win or lose—it's how you play the game." Will I sign up for next year's marathon? I'm thinking about it.

I can't resist leaving you with a very old joke:

"When my grandmother was sixty, her doctor suggested she get out and walk five miles a day. She's eighty-seven now and we don't know where the hell she is!"

~Bobbie Jensen Lippman

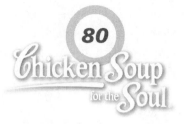

80

Heat Stroke

Never trust a private with a loaded weapon, or an officer with a map.
~Anonymous

Beyond being good for your health, being a runner will benefit you in ways you can't possibly foresee. With running comes energy and stamina on reserve, just in case you need it. Being a runner has helped me in countless ways, but none more than in PLDC.

Some people are gifted with sharp minds, and the ability to focus in very stressful situations. I was left entirely out of that exclusive club. In Platoon Leadership Development Course (PLDC), the Army's school for Noncommissioned Officers, I was forced to rely on running to save my military career.

Anyone who's ever enrolled at PLDC in Fort Dix, New Jersey will tell you that the toughest part of the class is the land navigation course. In order for a soldier to be deemed fit to lead, he or she must master reading and navigating with a map. Sounds easy, right? Perhaps for you. But for me, well, I don't always think things through, especially under pressure. As I crouched in the dirt on that hot July day down in the sprawling wilderness of Fort Dix, I knew I was in trouble.

Basic map reading is easy. Find the coordinates, line them up, bingo. There you are. Or at least, there's your 1,000-meter grid square. In order to be more accurate you must take your time and measure your grid square with a ruler. You must also shoot an azimuth with your compass, and be able to walk in a straight line over a long distance. There are various techniques that help you with these procedures, but I was in too big a hurry to use them. And so, after already wasting two of my allotted three hours to find my five checkpoints, all I could see was swamp, there were no landmarks in sight, and I hadn't seen any of the other 100 soldiers in an hour.

I was already sweating from the fatigues, boots, and heavy gear I was wearing, and from walking two miles in 90-degree heat into the middle of nowhere. Panic was just beneath the surface of my consciousness, and I fought to keep it down, but it just kept raising its head, and raising my blood pressure, making my heart slam in my chest. Anxiety was taking hold. I knew I had at least three miles to cover, and I had five checkpoints to find.

I tried to breathe evenly, pulled out my map. Okay. One good thing was that although my checkpoints were far apart, they were all fairly close to the highway that ran through Fort Dix. And that highway was long, and ran north to south on the border of my map. That meant that if I ran east long enough, I'd have to run into that highway eventually.

I began chugging along, fighting to find dry ground on which to run. Swamps were everywhere, and could sneak up on you if you weren't looking where you were going. I took deep, measured breaths, tried to find my natural rhythm. I checked my compass, kept heading east, and sure enough, began hearing cars. The highway lay before me. I ran up to the roadside, stopped to catch my breath. I only had a half hour left.

I began running hard down the side of the highway. Luckily it ran due south, so I didn't have to check my map. My back ached from the pull of my backpack straps, and my canteens banging against my sides. Onward I chugged, and after 10 minutes I could see my first checkpoint in the woods, 50 yards or so from the road. Four to go. The only problem was that I only had 25 minutes left. I knew many soldiers already had to be finished.

I began sprinting along my azimuth with wild abandon. When navigating over land with a compass, it is integral to know your pace count, and to count your paces. Otherwise you won't know how far you've traveled. Running wildly down the side of the highway,

I decided to abandon my pace count altogether. I was taking huge strides anyway. Which meant I'd have to be awfully careful about looking for my checkpoints.

I found my second checkpoint, and knew I'd have to turn into the woods. I had 15 minutes left. I hastily shot an azimuth that was nearly due west, noted on my map that I'd come across a road soon if I was headed in the right direction, and began an all-out sprint. I could hardly watch where I was going, because of the brambles I kept bursting through along my haphazard course. I put my Kevlar down and dug in, and suddenly I broke cover and hit the path I hoped to find. And before me was the third checkpoint. I wrote the number down. Two more to go.

I was sweating, panting, and my canteens were empty. Worse, I was beginning to feel a bit faint and nauseous. I felt the skin of my arm with my hand; it wasn't quite so clammy as before. I was beginning to show the first signs of heat stroke. Still, I had to keep on. I had 10 minutes left.

I shot a hasty azimuth from the bend in the path I was on, due south. If I ran true I'd hit one, then the other checkpoint, and if I really hustled I'd make it back in time. I hadn't really considered that: it wasn't enough to simply find one's checkpoints. You had to make it back too. I ran heavy, chugging my arms, my dummy M-16 swinging back and forth, clipping trees as I went. I stumbled upon my fourth checkpoint, hastily recorded it, and with not even enough time to check my watch I picked out a tall tree that was more or less due south and sprinted for it. I was heaving by this point, my clothes drenched, my skin eerily dry, though I'd been running for three hours straight in the hot sun, bundled up for 40-degree weather, as we all had to be. I crashed through a stand of pines, found my last checkpoint, and charged on, due south. I dropped a canteen, left it. I ran my heart out, even as my nausea increased and I panted like a heat-stricken dog. I finally saw a clearing ahead, broke out of the woods, and sprinted. I could see my fellow soldiers up ahead of me, could hear them yelling to me. I knew what that meant: there was still time. They wanted me to hurry.

I widened my stride and loped, putting one heavy boot before the other. I couldn't even hear them over my own slamming heart and riotous breathing. When I crossed the finish line and joined them, I'd had only a minute or so to spare. But I wasn't out of the woods yet, so to speak.

We were all organized into lines, and told to stand at attention while instructors looked over our maps and checkpoint lists to see if we found the right ones. But something funny was going on: I couldn't catch my breath. Ten minutes I stood there panting and heaving, and my lungs still thought I was running, apparently. I tried to focus on my breathing to even it out, but to no avail. My chest heaved and heaved. I felt my forehead, and it was dry. So were my hands. I was close to vomiting from nausea, and I was getting the chills. Which is odd in extreme heat. There was only one thing to do. I began to strip.

There was a female instructor that I didn't know leaning against the wall, and while everyone else was locked up tight at the position of attention, she saw me drop my rucksack and start taking off my shirt. She began to protest but I said two words that quieted her: "Heat stroke." I then took the canteen from the man's holster in front of me and drank it, took the canteen from the man behind me and dumped it on my head. They could have threatened me with discharge, and I wouldn't have stopped. Anything's better than getting heat stroke. In the end the instructors understood, simply watched with amused looks as I stole canteens from soldiers at attention and dumped them on myself. When I got to the front of the line my breathing had settled a bit, but I looked like hell. My shirt had been hastily buttoned back on, and I was soaked from head to toe, still panting, my face and arms striped with scratches from charging through the underbrush.

As the officer handed me back my test, which I passed, she said, "Damn, soldier. You look like hell."

"Yes Ma'am," I said. "Feel like it too." But I thanked God I was a runner.

~Ron Kaiser, Jr.

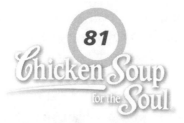

81

To Finish the Race

Good things come slow — especially in distance running.
~Bill Dellinger

'd moved to the back of throngs of shorts-clad humanity. "Excuse me, how fast do you run?" The answers ranged between eight- and nine-minute miles. Too fast for me. I kept slipping toward the back of the pack.

I've always wanted to be a fast runner. I'm not. I've tried speed drills, fartleks, you name it. I can't seem to break a ten-minute mile and on long runs I'm closer to twelve. You'd think this would embarrass me right out of running altogether. Nope. I still love running. On my own, training, I have no idea that I'm slow. I used to say dog slow, but my dog can run me into the ground. I don't like to insult her.

I used to weigh three hundred and twenty pounds. I don't anymore. Running is responsible for part of my weight loss. Slow I can deal with. It's better than being where I was — unable to walk up a flight of stairs.

I looked around. Nervous folks trying to look cool in their new clothes, race numbers pinned carefully. A group of women wearing tutus and tiaras danced around to my right. Nearby, what looked like a family surrounded a laughing woman who seemed to wear her bald head like a prize. This was my speed. I settled in to await the start of the race.

I nervously looked at a man to my right. "Have you run this before?"

He nodded. I figured he was too focused to talk. I bent down and retied my shoes for the eighth time that morning.

"I... run... a... lot." Slowly and carefully enunciated, the words plopped around me like the raindrops that began to ping the street. I looked up.

"I... like... run."

Half of the man's face formed words, half remained slack. His right arm plastered to his side, except for fingers that curled out in an odd direction.

I smiled and stood. "I like to run too."

Half of his face curled into a dreamy smile. Separated by many years and life experiences, we shared a moment of understanding. The struggle to run is worth it.

The gun banged in the distance, almost three blocks away. There was probably a countdown, but that far back in the pack, it was impossible to hear it.

Nothing happened. My end of the race always starts with a slow shuffle that eddies around, then sweeps you up and carries you along. "I don't know if I can do this." My voice cracked.

A woman dashed around us. "On your left." She surged through the crowd, a thoroughbred among Clydesdales.

"So... fast."

I smiled at the man to my right. I often start my races just like her. Moving around others. Fighting to be farther ahead. Forgetting that I am only racing myself. I often speed out of the gate and end up walking halfway through my races. Not today. Today I was going to stay at the back of the pack and run the entire distance. I'd trained for it. Prepared myself for this very race as if it was the only one. Ten miles. The longest race I'd run to date. I was going to triumph. I knew it.

The shuffle turned into a trot, then a jog. My companion fell behind me now. His shuffling gait distinctive and inexorable. Admiration filled me. I don't know if I would continue running if life handed me a hurdle so high.

Spreading out like wind-tossed leaves, runners headed into the first mile, settling into their paces. Each person looked determined and strong. The rain fell in hard drops that stung my skin. The effort already felt like too much. The miles stretched out in front of me, seeming to get longer with each step. I looked at my watch. Slower than I'd planned.

A hill defeated me into almost walking. Tears stung my eyes. "I am not going to walk. I can't walk." No matter how loud I said it, the desire to slow down and give my legs a rest became increasingly compelling. Head bowed, I crested a high hill plodding into a walk. I'd failed. I did not run the whole race. Why bother? What was the point of going on?

The man who'd suffered the stroke passed me. A smile on his face, determination in his gaze. His gait awkward but steady, he ran on. He was not calling a time out. "Come... on." His good arm gestured to me.

Yes, I am a slow runner. People wonder why I even bother. They can almost understand the running, but the reason I race eludes them. This man got it. He clearly saw what I did and shared my love. Sucking in a deep breath, I began to trot.

I finished one mile, then another. The last block, the last turn, the finish line and my family waiting for me in the rain. I'd done it. Ten miles.

"You're beautiful. Congratulations." My husband pulled me close and for once, I did not tell him he was wrong, or make a disparaging comment about my face and body. I accepted what he said. I was beautiful. As beautiful as all the grateful and exhausted people that crossed the line that day.

I watched my running companion shuffle across the finish line as a large group of people swarmed him. One man was his mirror image, probably his son. I gave him a thumbs-up and he waved in reply, then was swallowed by the joy-filled crowd. We'd done it. Finished the race. An outward symbol of an inner struggle. Medals clanged on many of the necks we passed, each a testament to an accomplishment.

~Nancy Liedel

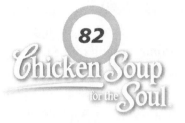

Mile 24

Most people run a race to see who is fastest. I run a race to see who has the most guts.

~Steve Prefontaine

Cheer for me... and I'll cheer for you! That's what his shirt said as he crossed us at Mile 24. This man, a stranger to us, was the first non-elite man to cross our station at the Boston Marathon yesterday and boy did we cheer. We cheered, hooted, hollered, jumped up and down and watched him do the same. As he passed us, he raised his hands to get the crowd even more excited (as if that was possible), clapped for us, and ran by, to finish the last 2.2 miles.

Soon, many more runners followed and we cheered just as hard for them as for the first. Many runners, young and old, passed us yesterday looking for inspiration. Some looked happy as we cheered. Some almost begged us with the look of pain on their face, and some actually asked, "Cheer for me?" And we did.

As the race wore on, many exhausted runners pushed their way to our station. It was clear that these people were going on pure hope. I could imagine that last year at this time, for whatever personal reason they had, they set their goal to run in the Boston Marathon and here they were at mile 24, still going.

Some of them got charley horses in front of us, and leg cramps, and overall exhaustion and started to walk. For these people we did all but run for them. We cheered louder, called out their names, or their numbers, we jumped up and down and pleaded with them to run...

and most of them did just that. We were fueled by our own ability to help them run, and so, even as we began to lose steam, and our own legs began to cramp from standing for so many hours, we stood and jumped and cheered and clapped. For the struggling runners, we went wild. We watched as they passed with dedications written on their jerseys—to charities or lost family members or diseases or their children. We watched as these people, these strangers, accomplished small miracles. And then, out of nowhere we saw (and heard) Team Hoyt approaching Mile 24. (For those of you who don't know about them, they are a father and son duo who have raced in over 900 events, including the Ironman.) Dick, the father (age 65), and Rick, his son (age 44), raced by us in their 25th Boston Marathon! Mile 24 was at the bottom of Heartbreak Hill so the momentum prevented Dick from raising his hands to us, so he zigzagged across the road, never once letting go of his son's wheelchair, to show his appreciation. Thank you Team Hoyt!

Our own runners stopped to hug their kids, enjoy jellybeans, thank the crowd, and then they were off again. These runners dedicated the race to a child who passed away from cancer, and we cheered each and every one of them on and through the finish line. One of them passed with "Pull" written on the front of his jersey and "Push" written on the back. The crowd went wild for this because they knew they were the ones pushing and pulling.

The day was filled with runners who ran on pure inspiration, and crowds who cheered on complete strangers. As we watched the last runners, it occurred to me that they were going to finish the race, not because they had to, but because they said they would. They set their goal and shared it with friends and family who they knew would offer positive reinforcement and inspiration. Most of the runners were not top athletes, and many of them were first-timers. They made up their mind, trained for it and kept telling people that they were going to do it. It's that simple. They did all the hard work and when they needed the push or pull to keep going, they didn't have to look any farther than to the sidelines where everyone wanted the best for everyone.

Remember the saying… "Runners just do it—they run for the finish line even if someone else has already reached it first."

~Christine A. Brooks

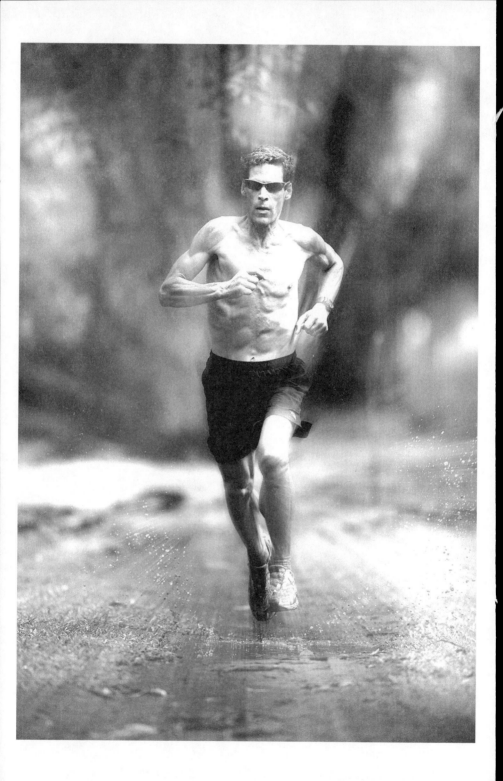

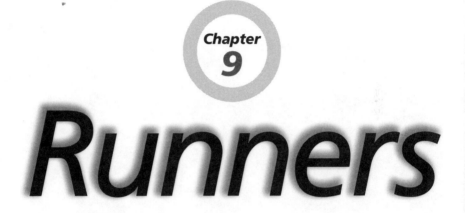

Chapter 9

Runners

Interesting Places

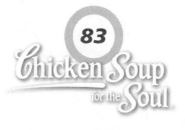

83

Push

A sign on the door of Opportunity reads Push.
~Author unknown

This is hard. Running across the country is hard. It's been seven months on the road. I've run the equivalent of 94 marathons. I'm getting tired, but I've been humbled.

Mountain ranges have tested my mental capacity to think positive. There is no way around the mountains. There is no way to dig a hole under them and excavate my way through. The only way is to go over these warriors that test my limits.

It is ironic that obstacles, those that are thrust in our faces, have an ulterior motive. That motive is to make us doubt ourselves, to raise the possibility of succumbing to fear, and to offer the option of quitting. I have no option but to take on these challenges. They are bigger than me and I need to find the strength within me to battle them. I cannot hit a wall and sit down. I must persist!

When you want something bad enough, that is the option you must give yourself—the only option: that you must persist. No matter what it takes, you will push through, climb every mountain in your own way, and come out a humbled, wiser, more appreciative and proud human being.

The last month in New Mexico has been... surprising. How do I put it? I've been in the state since October 2nd, exactly 31 days, and it has been surprisingly difficult to push on despite the enchanting culture and gorgeous landscapes. We have not had a homestay with a family in 31 days. Why is that? The land is sparse, and as one

New Mexican native put it, "people are hiding out… they like their privacy… they like their space and want to keep it." He jokingly continued, "What other state has more places named 'Outlaw Post' or 'Hide-Away'?!" (We have met many wonderful people. It's just that none of them have invited us to stay with them in their homes like most people have since Boston.)

Not being able to break bread with people makes me wonder. Why am I doing this? If there are no people, what is the point? But I know better than to let that thought effect my actions and plug up my forward-moving gusto. Again, it's another challenge, an instance that inspires a "what-the-heck-am-I-doing" moment.

But alas, there is no gain if you do not persist. If I break my foot, I will crawl. I will walk using a crutch. There is no quitting. If there are no people that want to help, I will move forward with the fuel people have added to the fire already over the past seven months on the road. There are a million reasons to keep going, and all the reasons to quit are the lazy ones.

I ran up that darn mountain with that blasting wind, and then felt proud. I flashed a big smile (literally) on a run during which I felt like a blob, and then felt stronger. I called a past host from Pennsylvania to say "hi," and then felt more connected to my mission and what this run is doing for people across the country. My point is to PUSH, however you can.

Stride on! One foot in front of the other. Find your inner strength. I keep telling myself these mantras. It will all be worth it. I want it badly enough. Do you want what you want badly enough? You should. That is the way it should be. Go get it… stride on!

~Katie Visco

Editor's note: This story was written during the seventh month of Katie's Run Across America, near Socorro, NM.

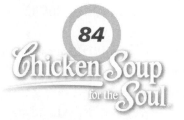

84

Women Can Run Too

There are victories of the soul and spirit. Sometimes, even if you lose, you win.

~Elie Wiesel

"Women can't run races," Muhammad said in French. "Girls, maybe. But not women and never mothers."

"I have three children and we ran 19 kilometers last Friday," I said in Somali. "Sign us up."

In Djibouti, a country the size of Massachusetts, running was reserved for the elite African men and French military. Three American women racing was unheard of.

"You speak Somali!" Muhammad said. "She speaks Somali. Sign them up."

As expatriate civilians, the three of us didn't belong to a Djiboutian running club or French military group. Muhammad insisted we were from Camp Lemonier, the American military base.

"We're mothers and English teachers," I said. "Not military."

"But you run."

"Yes, we do."

"You must be soldiers."

Finally he wrote our names down as members of the non-existent "Club American."

"May Allah give you a wonderful race and may you inspire Djiboutian women to run," he said. "The race will start at 3:30. Or 4:00. Or 4:30. Insha Allah." God willing.

Friday afternoon the other Americans and I arrived at Djibouti Telecom at 3:30, the hottest time of the day in one of the hottest countries in the world. At over 90 degrees, the day was considered cool by most and downright cold by others.

The Djibouti Telecom-sponsored race was 18K, but for the last nine years it had been 15K. T-shirts, the hand-painted banner draped over Djibouti Telecom's security gate and the newspaper advertised 15K. Spray-painted markings on the street read 18K. When I measured after the race, the total distance came to 18.6 kilometers.

The Djibouti National Team arrived and began their warm-ups with the graceful, powerful strides of the East African runner. I envied their speed and their shorts. As a woman in a Muslim nation, I wore long black pants and a baggy T-shirt.

After a quick trip to the "bathroom"—the dirt behind a metal wall blocking a construction site, we moved to the starting line. Alongside one hundred local participants (the newspaper reported 500) stood three American female civilians (the newspaper reported terrorist-fighting soldiers).

"I'll count to three," the head of the Djiboutian Sports Federation called out, "One…"

I glanced at the shoes around my Nikes and realized I was going to be lapped by men running in sandals and tennis shoes with the soles sewn back on.

"… two…"

There was a good chance I would come in dead last, but an image of Djiboutian women running with me one day made me lift my head high.

"… three!"

Within seconds, the Djiboutian men left us in their dust.

The first five kilometers looped around the Coke factory and the port where massive blue gantry cranes loomed above container ships. Mountains rose from across the Gulf of Tadjourah, dark shadows behind the brilliant dhows and white yachts. Men in fluorescent orange port uniforms glanced up from their tea, gaping as three women jogged by.

Soldiers and riot police blocked off the roads, holding back buses, taxis, goats and donkey carts. Spectators taking a break from repairing tires or handwashing laundry lined both sides of Rue d'Arta.

"Women... women... women."

Word spread down the street and people ran from restaurants, shops and their afternoon siestas and the throng swelled to four people deep.

The aroma of fresh-baked bread wafted towards us from behind fruit stands where bananas hung from ropes and watermelons were stacked ten high. Buyers and vendors stood in shocked stillness, their hands resting on an orange or holding open a plastic bag. As we neared Arhiba slum, the smell of bread was replaced by the stench of feces, urine and burning garbage.

"Les premières femmes!" The first women, we shouted, raising our hands in the air.

People cheered even though we were in last place.

We dodged potholes, sheep and across from Dar Al-Xanaan, the women's maternity hospital, my partners deftly leaped over the decomposing mass of a dead dog.

Beggar children climbed into the back of a lorry and chanted high-pitched, raucous songs, clapping in rhythm and squealing when I reached out for a high-five. Girls watched in awe and groups of boys ran alongside us until they were beaten back by the police.

With four kilometers remaining, I urged the other women, both stronger runners, to go ahead.

"You're the last one!" children called to me as I pressed on alone.

"You're going to die!"

"You're so tired!"

"You can't keep up with the men!"

"You're beautiful!"

"I know!" I shouted back to each one, alternating between Somali, French and English.

Encouragement came from the side of the road when an old man said in a low, serious voice, "You're doing *formidable*. Keep going."

I surged up the only hill in Djibouti, heading into the main market. Souvenir sellers hawked wares from Ethiopia and Kenya. Djibouti's main mosque, its white minaret stretching to the sky, was filled with men for evening prayers. Women clutched sacks of grain and bundles of cloth. Children with yellow jugs tied to their backs walked, bent over at the waist.

Everyone rose to their feet to clap and cheer. Policemen grinned and waved me on.

I was a champion. The entire market shut down to watch me run past. When has being in last place ever felt like bringing home the gold?

And then… a runner ahead. Then another. With one kilometer left, they were fading fast and I passed two Djiboutians, one because he stopped twenty yards from the finish line for a drink. I nearly collapsed across the finish line, third from last, third woman.

Before I could catch my breath, I heard my name called over a loudspeaker.

"Madame Rachel Jones!"

I waved my hand in the air and tried not to dry heave.

The head of the Sports Federation called me to the front steps of Djibouti Telecom where the ten top male runners stood with trophies in their hands and medals around their necks.

"Third place!" he called out and pressed a trophy into my trembling hand. I turned, shocked, and a camera flashed in my face. He motioned me to stand next to the elite men and called up the other women, first and second place.

The newspaper and television crew took footage of all the winners, three American nobodies and the Djibouti National Team. The men shook our hands and left with their awards.

The morning after the race my local neighbor asked if she could run with me once a week. It would be the first time she had run in her life. A week after the race as I drove along the port road, I passed two Djiboutian women jogging. Two weeks later three female university students joined me for laps at the track.

Smelling burning garbage and feces, dodging dead dogs, high-fives to beggars and being the third-fastest 18K female in the country.

But the reward I treasure most is the thought that perhaps I was part of inspiring Djiboutian women to run.

~Rachel Jones

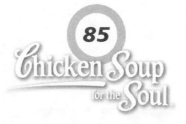

85

A New Road

There are clubs you can't belong to, neighborhoods you can't live in, schools you can't get into, but the roads are always open.
~Nike Corporation

Fifty-one days after my natural-childbirth-turned-induction-turned-Caesarean section, I started running again. I didn't get far—maybe a quarter of a mile—before I had to slow myself and the second-hand EZ Strider containing my sleeping son to a walk. And while a quarter of a mile is nothing to brag about for most runners, something in that moment made me feel like I was coming back: becoming myself again after seven weeks of feeling my old self—teacher, writer, runner—slip away, leaving behind nothing but a Baby-Feeding Machine.

I loved my son, of course, but during those seven weeks I felt heavy. With extra fat, yes, but also with sleep deprivation, with the nightmarish transformation of my beautiful non-medicated birth into a thirty-hour induction culminating in surgery and a painful recovery, and with the certainty that I would never be able to leave my house or cook my own meals again due to the seven-and-a-half pounds of humanity that had taken over my life. That's a lot to carry around, and with all of it weighing me down, it seemed unlikely that I would be running any time soon.

And yet, two days after my midwife gave me the all-clear to start exercising again, I placed Isaiah in the jogging stroller and went for a walk. We walked the next day, too, and the day after that. On that third walk, when Isaiah had nodded off on a quiet sunlit street, I started to run. I wasn't wearing the right shoes or the right clothes; the off-kilter stroller tugged me to the right with every step, and my lungs had no idea what had just hit them, but man, did I feel good. Lighter. Freer. A little more at home inside my own life than I had felt for a while.

It reminded me of Kansas. And Kraków. A year before Isaiah was born, my husband Matt and I had celebrated our wedding in Matt's birthplace of Lawrence, Kansas. I had been the one to suggest moving the wedding from my family's native New York to the less pricey, more laid-back Midwest, but I'll admit it was strange getting married away from home. I didn't know where to get my hair done or what the wedding traditions were; I had to depend on Matt and his family for all of that. The whole experience, though wonderful, gave me a fish-out-of-water feeling that I had never imagined as part of my wedding.

But while I couldn't give any of my guests driving directions, and I couldn't do more than imagine what a wedding reception in a barn would be like, most days I could run. I ran with Matt's brother Paul and sister Lisa near their parents' farmhouse, past wheat fields and old cemeteries. And I discovered something: running in a place makes it yours.

Away from home, when I put on those clothes christened with my sweat and pull on those grungy socks and shoes that countless miles have molded to my feet, it's like putting on my pajamas in a hotel room and plunking my slippered feet up on the furniture, like blasting the stereo and slipping into the bubble bath in a guesthouse. I'm telling everyone, "Yeah, I belong here. I'm comfy and I'm going to get comfier." When I hit my stride on a foreign footpath, I'm saying to that place, "Let's get to know each other, but let's not do it at arm's length. Let's take our hair down and forget the formalities. I'm going to act like I'm at home with you, and you'll treat me like an old friend. How about it?"

Fresh from our honeymoon, Matt and I boarded a plane to Kraków for my brother's wedding with maybe three Polish phrases under our belts. When we got there, we stayed at a hostel where we easily raised the average age by ten years. We couldn't have left our room without maps and phrasebooks any more than without our clothes. But I could still run.

My feet slapped cobblestones and made the side streets of Kraków mine. I wove around the grounds of Wawel Castle and made the castle mine. I circled the city center while shopkeepers opened their doors and waiters set up tables on the sidewalks, and I made that square mine. And yes, I got lost. But that was okay, too. Fumbling goes with the territory sometimes, and when I calmly turned to retrace my steps, I was telling Kraków, "No big deal. I belong here, and I'm going to keep acting like it. Thanks for the cool detour."

A few months later, back in New York, my brother-in-law Paul and I went for an eight-mile run along the Bronx River—my turf—on World Run Day. Soon thereafter I learned I was pregnant; then came the nausea, exhaustion, and weight gain that made running at first uncomfortable and eventually impossible. Almost a year later, while Paul completed his training for the New York City Marathon, I gripped the handle of that EZ Strider and spurted into my quarter-mile comeback. "Yes, I belong here," I was telling motherhood. "Good to know you."

~Marian Tascio Friedrichs

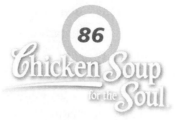

86

You Can Go Home Again

Youth is the gift of nature, but age is a work of art.
~Stanislaw Jerzy Lec

s my plane approached the outskirts of Warsaw, the rural landscape of farms and haystacks gave way to a collage of multi-colored roofs clustered around the jutting spires of the Palace of Culture, rekindling memories I thought had been extinguished. I pressed my hand to the cabin window, gaping through my fingers like the wide-eyed little girl who left Poland so long ago for a better life in America.

I thought I would never return to the Iron Curtain land of my youth. But here I was, forty-two years later, determined to run the Warsaw Marathon.

Once on the ground, I took a taxi to my hotel. Decades of capitalism had altered the city to such an extent I hardly knew where I was most of the time. An endless array of high-end department stores, wine merchants and fast food restaurants greeted me as my cabbie wheeled his Mercedes down the tree-lined avenue. I was both pleased and a little overwhelmed at the changes prosperity had wrought. Had I made a mistake in coming here?

As a fifty-something veteran of fifteen marathons, I knew my best performances were behind me. The Warsaw race was serious business, dominated by fast men with endurance, such as local hero Grzegorz Gajdus and the Kenyans, Richard Rotich and Reuben Toroitich. Who was I to run with the likes of them?

Two days before the race I picked up my entrant's packet in Stare

Miasto, a restored section of Old Town in Warsaw's historic district. Arriving at Castle Square, I saw the marathon festivities were already in progress. Local humanitarian Marek Szuster was running on a treadmill, trying to establish a new world record to raise awareness for sufferers of multiple sclerosis. Caught up in the moment, I found myself joining in as schoolchildren chanted, "Marek, Marek, Marek is our hero!" adding a silent chorus under my breath of, "Janine, Janine, will you be a zero?"

On Saturday, a day before the race, a host of volunteers served up a pre-marathon dinner in Podzamcze Park of pierogi, kielbasa and pasta with marinara sauce. It was all washed down by pitchers of carb-loaded beer, the runners' beverage of choice the night before the race in lieu of the usual vodka.

Marathon day was picture-perfect, encouragingly sunny and crisp, with temperatures in the low 50s. The race started in front of Castle Square, a picturesque spot at the entrance to Old Town. As I stretched and paced, the narrow cobblestone and brick streets reminded me of Paris' Latin Quarter. The cobbles were as picturesque as they were hard on the feet, as I would learn near the end of the race.

The starter fired his gun and the crowd erupted in cheers as we began our journey through history down a wide, smoothly paved street, shaded by tall buildings with flowers cascading from balconies.

Nearing the Palace of Culture, we passed the only palm tree in Warsaw, (plastic of course). The city center was a place of broad boulevards with sidewalks wide enough for cars to park three deep. The route took us past the museum home of Madame Curie, (Maria Sklodowska, to us Poles), then on to John Paul II Avenue and beside statues of Copernicus and Frederick Chopin. I felt small beside these giants of science, faith and art, as though I might be Thumbelina in gym shorts, running on an enormous postcard of Slavic culture and history.

As the sun rose higher above the skyline, the temperature rose with it. Schoolchildren dressed as clowns, fairies and princesses lined the streets, offering us drinks, fruit and chocolate and cooling our overheated bodies with wet sponges.

A little boy holding a bucket of water above his head offered to douse me. I answered his politely shouted, "Moge?" (May I?) with an equally respectful, "Nie!" A sweet offer but I didn't relish the thought of finishing the race in soggy shoes. Much to the lad's delight, I tossed him my gloves as I passed by. From the look on his face I may have created the first of many racing memories for a budding marathoner.

On the last leg of the race we crossed a bridge over the Vistula River with a panoramic view of the ancient city. The last four kilometers included a foot-pounding descent on a cobblestoned hill, leveling out along the river bank and finally a sprint to the finish in Podzamcze Park.

Nearing the end of my stay I managed a visit to the little village of Novogrod where I grew up. Strolling by the banks of the Narev River I happened to meet Marcin, a young man sporting a pair of running shoes nearly identical to mine. No sooner had we traded knowing looks than we simultaneously dug into our pockets and proudly displayed our finishers' medals. I could barely suppress a giggle as his eyes bulged and jaw went slack. "Yes, it's gold," I replied to the question he couldn't bring himself to ask. "I finished first place in my age group." He shouted to a group of friends and before I knew it I was a minor celebrity in the village I left so long ago. Basking in the warmth of their good wishes, I felt my eyes welling with tears.

My long overdue return to Poland had proven beyond a doubt that you can go home again.

~Janine Fleury

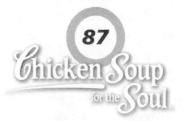

87

You Can Run,
But You Can't Hide

The secret of cross country is to do everything we do on the track and take it into the bush.
~Mike Koskei, former national coach of Kenya

"**D**o you think you'll pack shorts to run in?" Recently I'd received a string of messages from this strange girl who had found my blog online. At that point, we didn't really know much about each other, but it didn't really matter. We had one monumental thing in common: we were about to embark on an incredible journey as US Peace Corps Volunteers (PCVs) in the tiny, primarily Muslim, West African country of The Gambia, and we needed to know exactly what to fit into the two allotted suitcases we would live from for the next two years. After doing a little more research and discovering that a woman showing her knees in a village is akin to showing up to a dinner date topless, I decided that I would bring one pair of shorts for running in the "city" near the coast, but also a pair of three-quarter length synthetic work-out pants to be on the safe side. After all, everything I had read about The Gambia never failed to mention the hot season highs reaching 120 degrees in some parts of the country.

We arrived as Trainees to a large coastal town in The Gambia at the beginning of February, in the midst of the "cold season." The combination of an orientation session in blustery Washington, D.C. with thirty-six hours of travel left me and a couple of other Trainees anxious to expend some of the energy that had been accumulating for the past week. What better way to do that, while exploring our new surroundings, than to go on a run?

Along with a few casual runners like myself and Shorts Stranger, my group happened to include a triathlete and a guy who ran for Team Nike before coming to Gambia. I remember our first run vividly. A more experienced PCV offered to take us on a route she enjoyed when she came down to the Kombos, the semi-urban area near the coast. When Shorts Stranger and I showed up at the meeting spot wearing the exact same, single pair of shorts each of us brought, it was friends at first run, despite ultimately being placed on opposite sides of the country. It was 6 PM and approximately 90 degrees... cold season, huh?

I was perturbed by the ridiculously large quantity of sand on the roadside. I sought solace in the assumption that the surplus of sand was a result of the proximity to the beach and that once we moved to our villages, there wouldn't be as much. Obviously, I'd missed that National Geographic series on West African topography. But then we were taken down a path that placed the Atlantic Ocean in our periphery and as the sun began to set over the cliffs on which we were running, I knew this was one hobby not getting left in the dust.

Here is what it's like to be a runner in West Africa, more specifically, a young, white female in a reserved Muslim country. Imagine if you will, you are in a public place, perhaps a shopping mall or supermarket, with many people going about their purpose. But your purpose isn't to shop. Your purpose is to go for a run and you have no choice but to run around the store in front of all these people. This causes confusion among the shoppers, many of whom will choose the wrong brand of bread as a result of staring at you while you pass. What's more, every hundred meters or so, a dollar bill falls out from the wad of cash you forgot to remove from your pocket. Each time, without fail, a handful of shoppers make it their mission in life to get your attention by shouting "Runner!!! Heyyyyy, RUNNER!!" the only obvious name which represents who you are to them. They will shout this over and over, whether you acknowledge them or not.

On top of that, some wise guy decides he's going to recreate that running scene in *Forrest Gump* and before you get the chance to turn down his question to join you running, he's trotting along beside you, asking "You a'right, mate?" and "From which country?" However, some of the shoppers think what you are doing is equivalent to saving small children from a burning building, so they take it upon themselves to be your personal cheerleader, shouting such phrases as "Keep it up, boss lady," "Strong girl," and my personal favorite, "Champion sport woman!"

In the villages where most PCVs serve it is almost unheard of to see a woman running. Women pound rice and millet with mortars and pestle the size of livestock, with babies strapped to their backs. They wash basin after basin of their family's clothes by hand, each bucket of water arduously fetched. They cook all the meals from scratch, hand filleting boney fish upon boney fish after 20 minutes of sifting through the previous day's pounded rice to remove unwanted debris, but not before chopping firewood. The fortunate girls get to attend school in addition to the aforementioned. They don't run for pleasure or exercise. Running is something only boys do, most likely wearing plastic jelly sandals, not even proper tennis shoes, when training for football.

Despite the Peace Corps protocol of placing each volunteer in separate villages to work with host country counterparts, I managed to maintain a series of running partners. During our first three months of language, culture and technical training, before swearing in as a volunteer and moving to a permanent site, I lived in the same village as Team Nike. We stayed in separate compounds with Mandinka host families, one of the predominant Gambian tribes. One of the first Mandinka phrases Team Nike and I learned, besides "It's hot" and "My stomach is paining me," was "I'm going running." Our evening runs into the African bush became somewhat of a therapy session in which we contemplated our new environment while challenging homesickness and the struggle of maintaining our American identities.

Nothing brings you closer to a running partner than amoebic

dysentery, at which point we would once again take advantage of our newly acquired language skills, and make light of our unusual situation. When I moved to a larger urban town at the start of my placement, I began running with the PCV whose job I took over, as she had decided to remain in Gambia for a few more months in order to work with another organization. Unwanted attention in that town was much more rampant than in the smaller villages, especially with the excitement of seeing not one, but two white females race by on the main road. Once again, though, time spent in motion together proved fecund, as we discussed relationships, developments and the bureaucracy behind the NGO with which I was now working.

On the other end of the spectrum, running in the Kombos was a bit different than running in village. In addition to the young boys who think it is the most entertaining thing to tag along with you, older men see it as an opportunity to "make a friend." One thing I have yet to mention about Gambia is its disreputable sex tourism industry. Oh yes! For a small price, even you can have your very own "bumster," a young male escort whom women will pay to accompany them on their vacation, who will serve as your personal tour guide, and show you a very intimate side of the Smiling Coast, a nickname given to Gambia by the Ministry of Tourism.

Apparently, bumsters also like to run. I mean, besides doing push-ups and callisthenic exercises in very little clothing on the beach, how else are they going to attract the middle-aged ladies? So, every once in a while, I would get my very own personal running buddy, in the form of a bumster. I never could quite tell which was more aggravating: those big, buzzing flies that also accompanied me, or the relentless bumsters.

Why did I run? Why did I put up with the constant stares and frequent shouting of "toubab," a West African reference to a person with my pigmentation? Why did I tolerate unwanted running partners and an endless sea of sand, all under a sweltering sun? Because not too much compared to watching that sweltering sun melt behind a shimmering, rust-colored savanna in village and, ultimately, the vast, azure-hued Atlantic. Because living thousands of miles away from home was no reason to stop logging hundreds of miles. Because I was a runner before and aspire to always be. And, because sometimes you just have to show a little knee.

~Courtney Gilman

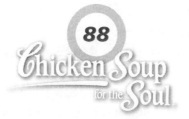

88

The Granddaddy

I feel like a Bull Moose.
~Theodore Roosevelt

I can't believe I'm in Alaska! I'm running the Campbell Creek Greenbelt, my steps as light as my heart. The paved trail snakes through woods of swamp spruce and birch. The air is fresh from a light morning rain, with temperatures in the upper 60s, warm for June. Birds chirp high overhead. How good can life get?

I'm visiting a friend for a week, and he's dropped me off to run this gorgeous trail while he works at his office. I'm hoping to add to the list of wildlife I've seen so far: the mountain sheep my friend and I spotted on a hillside on the road from Anchorage to Portage Glacier, a bald eagle that soared above us as we hiked the Coastal Trail, king and silver salmon we saw fishermen catch as they stood shoulder to shoulder along the bank of Ship Creek in downtown Anchorage.

Today I'm hoping to see a moose. Sometimes, I'm told, one can look across meadows and see the females, called cows, grazing. The term "cow" delights me. I'm sure they'll look nothing like the herds of dairy cows I pass on runs in rural areas of Oregon. I'm told the cows seldom venture close to the trail, and aren't aggressive unless someone gets between one of them and her baby; that Bull Moose are never seen on the trail.

Sounds good to me; interesting, but safe.

High with the thrill of it all, I round a corner and almost into the side of a moose. Not a female across a meadow. A huge Bull Moose standing where the woods open into a grassy space. My nose is at most two feet from his enormous side.

I freeze. My chest constricts. My heart beats triple time. What happened to safe?

Seconds pass. The moose doesn't twitch a muscle. Could it be a statue? I see no movement of breath. Whew. I might have known. The beast is too big, the rack too broad to be real. I've seen moose heads mounted on stone fireplaces in lodges and they aren't nearly as huge as this one. It makes sense to have a statue of the state animal of Alaska in this park, along a trail dozens of people use daily. Ah well, a statue of a moose is better than no moose at all.

The sculptor has done an amazing job. I can almost see the individual hairs on the giant body. My heart rate slowing, I reach my hand out to touch the animal's metal side.

The statue turns its head toward me, ever so slightly, and rolls a huge, brown eye.

It's real. My heart pounds. Goosebumps rise along my arms. My mind spins an image of that rack crushing my body.

I slide one foot backward, then the other. Step by slow step I move away from the Bull Moose.

When I've backed around the corner, I turn and sprint the opposite direction. I've never run so fast.

Two young men on mountain bikes ride toward me on the trail. They look to be about twenty, the age of my oldest son. I motion for them to stop. "There's a moose up there, a big bull. You might want to turn around."

They look at each other, then at me, and smile, the kind of slightly patronizing smile one might offer a cowardly, middle-aged woman. "Don't think we'll worry about it," one says. "We see them all the time." And off they ride.

I run on, still thinking of that huge head turning toward me. That rack the size of my dining room table. I've run just a few more minutes when the two young men appear at my side, this time going my direction. "We thought we'd leave the trail to him," one calls out as they pass, this time a trace of sheepishness in his smile.

What an experience. Running, my mid-life passion, has given me not only increased bone density, muscle strength, and endurance, but also the opportunity to meet the granddaddy of all Bull Moose. I hug the image of the moose to me as I slow to a jog and continue my run.

~Samantha Ducloux Waltz

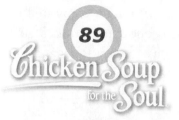

Footprints around God's World

It's elevating and humbling at the same time. Running along a beach at sunrise with no other footprints in the sand, you realize the vastness of creation, your own insignificant space in the plan, how tiny you really are, your own creatureliness and how much you owe to the supreme body, the God that brought all this beauty and harmony into being.
~Sister Marion Irvine, 2:51 PR and 1984 U.S. Olympic Marathon Trials qualifier

"You're going to wear that out in public? You must be jokin'!" six-year-old Helen Rafferty asked me in a lilting Irish brogue as she watched me unpack my running shorts and tank top. I could tell that her mother, standing near the lace curtains, was thinking the same thing.

Oh great! If they really don't wear running gear here in the Emerald Isle, then I'm going to have to spend a titanic amount of my Guinness money on a sweat suit. At least then I won't stick out while running the next few months.

And that's just what I did. Like a banshee, I scoured Dublin that fall day in 1986. I finally found a turquoise warm-up suit. It wasn't my style, but at least now I was ready to hit the cobblestones. Even though Dublin had a small marathon at that time, I deduced that the Irish hadn't been bitten by the running bug. It seemed like I was the only runner out there during the entire semester I studied abroad.

And so it didn't really matter what running gear I wore, because regardless of what I threw on, I stuck out like a fitness freak anyway.

I found it curious that the running craze hadn't reached this island yet. Jogging had been so popular in America ever since *Rocky* hit the big screen in 1976, when I was ten and had become a runner myself. Even on cold days a person couldn't drive around my home state of Minnesota without seeing people running through neighborhoods, along the banks of the Mississippi or on paths around our numerous lakes. I pondered: Had the running craze bypassed only Ireland, or had it leapfrogged the entire world, only to be popular in the United States?

It's been twenty years since I first wrestled with that query. I have traveled the world with my husband due to incentive trips he is blessed to win. In the early nineties, at our vacation destinations, the only people "hitting the road" were my triathlete husband, some of his American co-workers and yours truly. The locals looked upon us as alien creatures come to seize control of their sidewalks, paths and streets.

The place I got ogled the most was Vienna, Austria in 1995. I had an hour to kill before my presence was expected at a meeting, so I laced up my sneakers and decided to run through Stadtpark. During my 3-mile course I didn't encounter any other runners. I noticed the same phenomenon on other days. Obviously, the jogging bug hadn't bitten in this part of the world either. As I rounded the Johann Strauss monument, I noticed a very gentrified man staring at me. I recalled reading a book before our trip that stated the Austrians were in the midst of a national decrease in births. I read that there would not be many expectant women or babies in Vienna, and the author was right! I'm sure I looked rather goofy to this dapper gent as I approached him in a bright pink T-shirt and matching Spandex shorts. I'll admit, it wasn't the prettiest set of running clothes I owned, but it was the only thing I could find to fit over my large, pregnant belly. So you see, I looked very much the outsider to him... an expectant mom and a jogger all rolled into one!

My husband and I have trotted God's globe from sea to shining sea on these business trips. From the lakes of Minnesota to the hills of Hong Kong, we've created extraordinary memories along happy trails. When we commune with nature in this remarkable way, we feel God's pleasure. As we've carried forward (even after my husband's diagnosis of rheumatoid arthritis in his late thirties), we've wondered: If running is so beneficial, why aren't people all around the world getting hooked on this exuberant sprint for life? Even my husband's specialists are saying how healthy exercising is for everyone: to persevere and just do it!

And so, we do keep running all over the place. If we're not dashing after our seven kids, we're making tracks along the beaches of Mexico or the mountains of New Zealand. Why shop in different nations when there's so much glory to see as we run?

It finally happened in Barcelona in 2000. My husband accompanied me as I went for a slow run (more like a waddle since I was eight months pregnant) and we actually saw Spanish people out there jogging along the sea! I could tell they were avid runners because of the athletic gear they had on. It was wonderful. The running fever wasn't just in America anymore. And further proof that the Spanish attitude had reconditioned was the fact that when we neared the hotel, after our morning jog, instead of strange looks from the doormen, we were handed a cold bottle of spring water from an ice bucket and a moist towel with which to wipe our sweat. Now there are road races all over Europe. There are marathons in Africa and Antarctica.

In a few months, my husband of seventeen years and I will travel to Ireland with his company. I'll pack my tank top and running shorts, and not the turquoise sweat suit (I left that in Ireland back in 1986). I can jog in my regular running clothes because I know I won't get odd looks from the locals; Ireland has joined the U.S. in a running craze. The Dublin marathon has grown from 2,100 participants its first year in 1980, to 11,000 entrants this year. In fact, when we were visiting the Emerald Isle in 2004 we actually came across a bloke training for the Dublin marathon. This young man left hobbled prints by the River Liffey; he had pulled his Achilles tendon. But the thrill of the upcoming race was evident in his freckled face. I noticed he was wearing soccer gear, but heck… he was a runner!

~Kathryn Schneeman

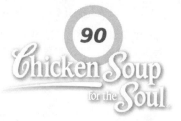

90

Each Step an Offering

Take a breath of the new dawn and make it a part of you.
~Hopi Proverb

Inspiration

It's 1:30 in the morning, only a quarter mile into what is planned to be a 44-mile day, and I have already stripped down to my shorts and T-shirt. The Colorado River snakes its way through this canyon 5,000 feet below me. Moving over stone, my shadow keeps me company as my feet crunch down the South Kaibab Trail. I remind myself of the Hopi Indians, a Puebloan people who live nearby, and their belief that running can be a form of prayer. Each step is offered as a sacrifice to a loved one, and in return they ask the Great Spirit to match their strength with some of His own. I have never attempted such a big run, but motivated by my mother's recent victory over cancer, I am inspired to try the Hopis' way, offering each of my steps as a sacrifice to my mother's renewed health, with the hope of better understanding my experience of facing the unknown.

Preparation

Getting ready for a long run is straightforward. I increase my mileages, test my gear, familiarize myself with the route, and gather the proper foods to fuel my efforts. I ran throughout the spring, visiting beautiful places and accumulating big miles as I anticipated my pilgrimage. Despite my training, I felt my confidence swallowed by the Canyon as I approached its rim. Could I pull this off? Is this what my mom felt when she was diagnosed? Does our preparation ever match our challenges?

The Power of Community

When illness arrives it is easy to feel alone. Looking beyond our sense of isolation, we recognize groups of people who share our experiences. Heading alone into the Canyon, I was surprised to see another headlamp illuminating the trail a few switchbacks below me. When I caught up I was greeted with a friendly "Good morning." My loneliness evaporated; other people were on this path. Each time I had an encounter it refreshed my sense of shared mission and community.

Where are My Boundaries?

My first big landmark was the Colorado River. I glimpsed it as I descended, a silver ribbon defining the canyon bottom. Without its presence, my plunge would have felt like a tumble into nothingness. I remembered my mother deciding which doctor appointments were significant, which treatments would mark her progress. Finding ways to segment our experiences, we can handle overwhelming tasks. Inspired by what we have accomplished, we can face what lies ahead. Crossing the river I knew that one small part of my adventure was complete and I would now begin my 14-mile, 6,000-foot climb up to the North Rim.

Beauty Everywhere

Passing silently through Phantom Ranch on the north side of the river, I felt like the phantom himself. I was solidly entering the meditative mind and flowing awareness that running brings. Night-blooming flowers laced the air with perfume and iridescent insects flitted about in my headlamp's beam. Bright Angel Creek rushed invisibly past me on its way to the Colorado River. As stars began to melt away into the dawning sky, I found that unlike my experience heading into the Canyon, I was alone. I imagined my mother finding herself in the dark hours of a sleepless night, achy from chemotherapy, having to source the beauty of her life, the distant love of her friends and family to get through those times.

Illumination

Although morning brought with it stunning sunshine, temperatures dropped as I neared the North Rim. Ponderosa pines and aspens slept; the North Rim was not yet open for the season. As I lay on my back gnawing on a Lärabar smeared with Hammer Gel, feet propped up against a rock, I took a moment to reflect on my journey. I reminded myself that halfway is just that, exactly as far from the beginning as from the end. I recalled the celebration my parents had after reaching chemotherapy's midway point. Does completing half our task truly mean we will be able to finish it? An energizing breath followed my sigh of relief and I packed up to cross the canyon again.

One More Time

Gazelle-like, I bounded down the North Kaibab trail. Tackling this, the longest leg left in my journey, I considered that I had already covered 22 miles and experienced 11,000 feet of elevation changes. My mom must have had moments of total inspiration; getting good test results as cancer withered and died in the face of chemotherapy had certainly provided feelings of fearlessness. I had my reflective parasol anchored to my shoulder strap, my iPod pumped Abba into my ears, and I took time to appreciate that I was passing through one of the greatest places in the world. In the same moment I was aware that the temperature was approaching the predicted 102 degrees, I would soon be surpassing my longest training run mileage, and my food was beginning to repulse me.

Times Change

Passing through Phantom Ranch again was now a social event. Campers finishing breakfast seemed surprised to see me as I trotted across the Canyon for a second time. These people were not like the hikers with whom I had earlier shared my path. They reminded me of the caring people who offered, "Oh, I am so sorry to hear about your mom's illness," or the acquaintances who tried to show compassion, though ultimately felt uncomfortable dealing with the dark specter of cancer. Their support was mixed with a sense of relief that for now, they would only have to visit with suffering, not actually be its host. A cold green river had replaced the silvery ribbon I crossed eight hours ago and my pace slowed as I ran along its shore.

Will This Ever End?

At Indian Gardens I broke down and vomited my last energy bar and most of my water onto the hot sand. Though I shared the cottonwood tree's shade with other travelers, no one said anything about my condition. I had to accept that a journey's end is a definite place and I was not yet there. Eventually I would be able to mark the completion of my quest, but my mother's journey could have numerous finish lines. Cancer might find new hiding spots, allowing her to slow down and walk for a stretch; however, her race might have to be run again. Feeling alone and unable to completely reenergize, I let the nausea pass and then got up to finish my prayers.

Back Where I Started

Fortunately, the people in my life who have dealt with cancer have all outrun their sickness. The difficult journey forever changes their lives. Eventually, their suffering gives way to renewed health and life continues. During my run through the unknown each step had been an act of gratitude, an offering to the Great Spirit. As I surveyed the Grand Canyon from its South Rim, it was clear to me that life is just a series of journeys, one linked to the next, each ultimately bringing me a little closer to where I started and each one leaving its imprint on my life.

~Eli Shostak

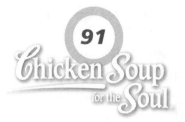

91

The Broken Toe

Giving up is your brain's idea. Ask yourself, who's in charge here?
~Phil Whyman

week before traveling to Baffin Island in Canada's Arctic in 1990 to run my twentieth marathon in a tiny mining village called Nanisivik, a race that I knew an ordinary runner like me had a chance of winning, I broke a toe. The first thing I thought was, "Oh good, I don't have to race."

After thinking long and hard about that I wondered if I had a fear of success and this was my way of dealing with it. And then I wondered how often I'd experienced this in my life.

I could have backed out but I would have lost most of my travel fee so I decided to go anyway and see how I felt. Twenty-six point two miles... what could go wrong? Several days of treatment and advice later, I wanted to give it the old college try. With the help of a small machine I borrowed that sent electrical currents through my throbbing toe and helped me deal with pain each day, I decided I could run with it bandaged.

The July Nanisivik Marathon was one of those races people said "You have to do" and that I should "Plan on adding on 20 or more minutes" to my best marathon time because of the terrain, the gravel road, the big hill at the end and the self-serve water stations. This event also had a 10K, 32K and double marathon, known as an "ultra-marathon" or "ultra."

At the airport an "ultra" veteran asked me which race, the marathon or double marathon, I was going to run. I proudly replied, "the marathon," to which he said, "oh, the wimp run." My first introduction to ultramarathoners!

The flight over Baffin Island was stunning—rough coastline, hundreds of islands flanking it, snow in places and a few mountains. Between the geography and a broken toe this was going to be an adventure like no other marathon.

Our group of 120 runners was housed in miners' homes and dorms for five days but ate and socialized at the community centre, the hub of mining life, where we gradually became a "family." Even the ultramarathoners talked to us marathon wimps! In between the fun stuff I diligently tended to my toe three times a day.

The day before our race, organizers bused us all to a desolate point we'd be passing the next day where a huge mound of rocks, or a "cairn" was placed lovingly by locals in memory of Terry Fox. My inspirations to run years prior were Terry Fox, the one-legged Canadian who, in 1980, ran halfway across Canada before succumbing to the cancer he thought he had beaten, and my mother, who struggled with cancer that same year. Ten years later I was in the Arctic the day before a marathon thinking of them again. Needless to say, I was moved by the northern minister (himself one of the runners) who led us in prayer, meditation and "Godspeed" in our event the next day.

That evening was the 10K, one of the highlights of the year for the locals. We veteran runners cheered the loudest at the finish line as the "weekend warriors" gasped in victory across the finish line and dozens of little Inuit kids ran themselves ragged to finish. Everyone was a hero that night.

Our race day route started in Arctic Bay, an Inuit village at sea level 20 miles from Nanisivik, plodding along gravel roads that meandered through what I'd liken to "moonscape," it was so bleak, rocky and lifeless. Our roads rose to altitudes of 1,000 feet above sea level in several places so it wasn't easy. Lifeless it was, yet there was an ethereal beauty to it too. Now I understood how people could misjudge distance with no landmarks to gauge it by.

My broken toe ached throughout the race in spite of the aspirin

I took halfway through. I planned to walk or stop if it got too painful, but until then I was in good enough shape to keep pace with the leader. How exciting was that—maybe I was going to throw off my "fear of success" mantle. I kept trying to psych out the leader by reminding him I was running with a broken toe. It didn't work!

We runners are used to having water handed to us in races but "water stations" at this race (and ultramarathons in general) were a jug of water and stack of cups on the ground—we were to help ourselves at each stop. Needless to say this slowed us all down a bit but we found it helped to stop together and take turns serving each other.

Course elevation jumped up and down but close to the village of Nanisivik and the finish line, it was an up section, rising to 1000 feet above sea level. At the 20-mile mark (32K) we ran past the finish line (which was such a tease to be so close) to the infamous "crusher" downhill portion. We knew it was coming—five kilometers (three miles) downhill, around a massive storage facility at the shoreline and then back up five kilometers—but it didn't mean we liked it. What twisted mind planned this route? What twisted minds were running it?

Oddly enough the long downhill that hurt my quad muscles and made the way back up really tough didn't affect my toe any more than it was already throbbing. But it was heading uphill that my first-place running compadre and I parted ways since I couldn't get anything else out of my legs. One more person passed me in that stretch and I finally hobbled to the finish line in third place overall to the cheers of hundreds of spectators. Talk about amazing hospitality—most of the spectators were local mine workers and Inuit residents and they all treated us like visiting dignitaries.

My broken toe was quite swelled and sore by the end of the race but ice packs, electric current and aspirin helped somewhat. I wasn't in great shape to play baseball that night at 2 AM—we were, after all, in the land of the midnight sun—but did anyway just to see the sun at that time.

Did I learn anything from my "run a marathon with a broken

toe" experience? Yes, I promised myself I'd never let fear of success get in my way again. I learned that I had a lot of determination, that I was "gutsy," that I wouldn't want to live on Baffin Island and that bacon for breakfast is good anytime but particularly in the Arctic after a marathon.

~Michael Brennan

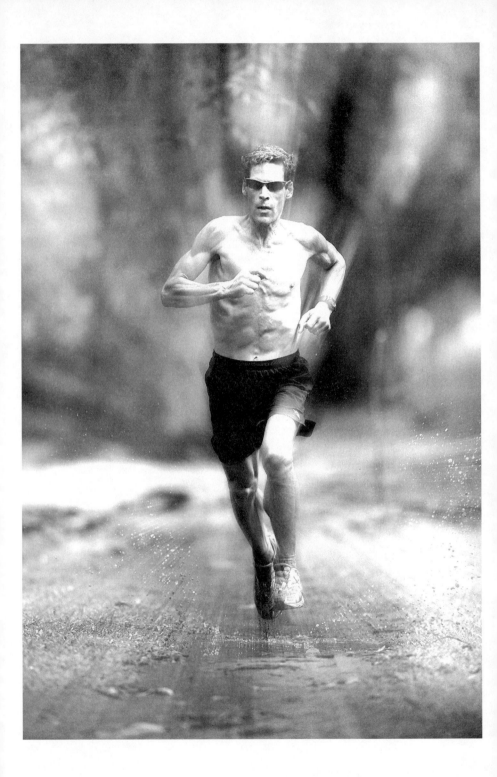

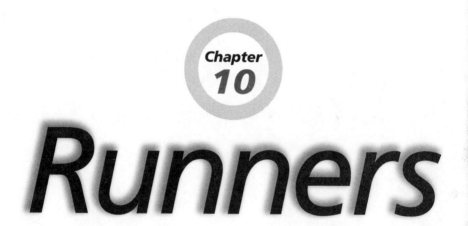

Chapter 10

Runners

Moving on to Triathlons

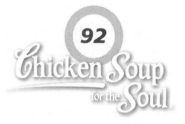

92

Ironman

I can be changed by what happens to me. But I refuse to be reduced by it.
~Maya Angelou

started running when turning forty, because who doesn't need something dramatic and studly when turning forty? Now I was turning fifty and set my sights on the Ironman Triathlon, because there are few events studlier than the 2.4-mile swim, 112-mile bike ride, and full marathon of an Ironman and who doesn't need something dramatic and studly when turning fifty?

While running, I earned amputee world records in distance and sprinting, but the records fell, as they always do, to younger, faster amputee women. I wanted a record I wouldn't lose. If I succeeded in being the first female leg amputee in the world to complete an Ironman, I would always be the first.

I called Lisa, my training partner of eight years, because I'm a relational gal and couldn't even think of training for Ironman by myself.

"Lisa, what do you think about doing Ironman?"

"What do I think? I think you don't know how to swim and you're terrified of the water."

"Well sure, but you can help me with that, can't you? You've been an amazing swimmer since you were a toddler."

The phone went silent. Then, "My swim career peaked before I graduated from the first grade, but no matter. I'm happy to help you with swimming. You can help me with the bike. I'm in!"

We chose the Madison Ironman, even though it had a killer

bike course, because it was close enough that our families could be there and the September temperature would probably be on the cool side. Weather plays a huge role in my ability to manage a race; heat and humidity affect how my prosthesis fits and how much pain I'll have.

That summer was cool for training but then unfortunately morphed into an autumn scorch. As Ironman Sunday approached, the prediction was for temps in the upper eighties with high humidity.

Prior to a race, I think anything's possible. I might have the best race of my life, or I might "crash and burn." Since I tend toward grandiosity, I usually anticipate having the best, but that morning, sitting on the banks of Lake Monona, my stomach churned. I didn't remember ever being so scared before a race. Not even the Paralympics. There's a special kind of stress with uncharted territory, in trying to be the first. Belatedly, I wondered why no amputee woman had ever completed an Ironman. I called upon my mantra from my first marathon: have fun with the day, focus on doing the best I could, be grateful for the opportunity to even be out there.

Maliq, my twelve-year-old son, a jock since he could walk, hugged me hard. "Mom, you are so gonna rock this course."

My husband Jeff, witnessing my fear, seemed a little less certain of my rocking anything, although he would feel it disloyal to doubt my ability.

Lisa and I entered the water as the sunrise lit up the sky. This would be the first race in which we would be racing as the sun came up and, if all went well, when the sun went down.

The horn blew and we and two thousand other swimmers were off. Arms and legs mashed, fighting for space before finding rhythm. I thought it encouraging that I didn't drown and sent out a silent "thank you" to the inventor of the wetsuit.

Once in the swim-to-bike transition, I grabbed my bike from its rack and ran the length of the parking lot, holding onto the seat post. Of the entire Ironman, this was my favorite moment, because not even most bipeds can run, full-out, steering from the seat post. I met Jeff by the exit so I could switch from my run-leg to my bike-leg.

On the second loop of the bike course, I passed through what looked like a battlefield, two-wheeler casualties strewn everywhere. The heat and wind were claiming an excessive number of racers. I then rode the course so conservatively that a gray-haired volunteer at the final water stop scolded me.

"You look really good."

"Thanks!"

"No, you look too good. Pick it up a little."

Had to be a coach; who else would admonish me for looking good?

I flew past Lisa a couple of miles before reaching transition. I was concerned; I shouldn't have caught her, because she had been so far ahead in the swim.

In the bike-to-run transition, I had stomach cramps, the back of my knee was rubbed raw from my prosthesis, and I was lightheaded, which reminded me to take salt tablets. I waited for Lisa and unfortunately when she arrived, neither one of us was thinking clearly enough to assess her condition. Lisa is a tiny woman, but later one of our friends said she had looked pregnant.

The beginning of the run in an Ironman is brutal. After so many hours going in a circle, legs have a hard time adjusting to the up and down of running. I ran. I walked. I stopped to fix my leg. Lisa and I lost each other.

The heat was unrelenting. I finally saw Jeff and Maliq a few miles from the finish line.

"Where's Lisa? I haven't seen her in hours."

"Honey, she's in the hospital," Jeff said.

"No!" Tears started. "What happened?"

"She lost consciousness when she saw us at the half-marathon point. The medics thought she was dehydrated but Mark called from the hospital. She's hyponatremic; her kidneys stopped processing fluids."

Jeff took my face in his hands. "Linds, look at me! She's going to make it; she would want you to finish this thing."

In that moment of perspective, the Ironman became "this thing" and I just wanted it to be over.

Maliq tried to help.

"Mom, let's run up this hill together."

I re-focused. "Darlin', these legs have no more 'run' in them."

But as we came up to the last hill, my feet ran on their own.

"Mom, you're a beast!"

When you're an almost fifty-year-old mother, there's little sweeter than hearing your teenaged jock son call you a beast.

The announcer screamed into the microphone, "Folks, cheer in the first amputee woman in the world to get here! Lindsay Nielsen, you are an Ironman!"

I cried. Maliq cried. Jeff cried, and people I had never met cried. I had done it and I knew, despite my disappointment that Lisa wasn't with me, it would be an accomplishment I would keep close forever.

We called Mark. Lisa survived, but she had nearly died that day.

Once back at the motel, my husband gingerly lowered my cramping body into the bathtub. I smelled like a neglected pig barn.

"I never need to feel this bad again. Maybe I'm a one-Ironman person."

A look of hope sidled across Jeff's face. Everything hurt, even my lungs and my tongue. Abs cramped with a ferocity that prevented me from standing up straight. My leg was rubbed raw in places and abrasions had opened up under my jog-bra. I felt like a human Velveteen Rabbit, full of bald spots.

Waking after a few hours of painful sleep, I started planning.

"When I do another Ironman…"

Whatever whisper of hope Jeff had dissipated into the stale air-conditioned room. He looked over at me with resignation on his face; we had been together for thirty years.

"Linds. I know you can't help yourself, but I'm tired. Give me a day, maybe even a week, and then you can have at it, and I'll be right there."

What would any of this be without family and friends?

As Lisa and I move through our fifties, we're looking for a new adventure, because who doesn't need something dramatic and studly when facing their sixties?

~Lindsay Nielsen

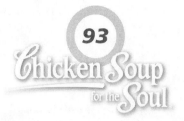

93

The Terror of Tri

Always do what you are afraid to do.
~Ralph Waldo Emerson

The second I hit the water, I knew I had made a mistake. There were about two hundred swimmers all diving in the lake at the same time, kicking off the first leg of our triathlon. We were indiscernible in black wetsuits and gray swim caps and kicked so much water that you couldn't see anything that wasn't right next to you. My wetsuit sucked against my stomach, keeping me from taking any deep breaths. The little air I took in was mixed with green water. I tried to hold my breath and swim underwater but the green murkiness blinded me. I could feel people swimming over the top of my legs and I knocked into someone with every attempted stroke. Panic quickly set in. Even though I was only thirty feet out, I knew I couldn't touch bottom, couldn't breathe, and couldn't see. This is how people drown.

I looked over the top of the other swimmers toward the rescue boats and saw they were too far out to save me if I went under. I considered swimming toward the boats to ask to be pulled in. All the training I had done in the last twelve weeks had not prepared me for this.

All this madness had really started three months previously. I had finally decided to train for a triathlon because I needed more motivation to stay fit. Competing in a triathlon terrified me and fear is a powerful motivator. I had been thinking about competing in a triathlon on and off for the past three years, but I thought I had talked myself out of it due to my fear of drowning or being hit by a car while biking.

It started from an innocent conversation. My roommate and I were commiserating about how our ambition level had dropped off with regard to exercise. Losing weight was no longer enough of a motivator, and I told her I needed something to work for. And then those words that I had never dared say out loud came out, "We should compete in a triathlon." She quickly squelched the idea for her, but something about saying it out loud to someone cemented the idea into a goal for me.

I had just over three months to train for the next triathlon in my area. I bought the aptly titled *The Complete Idiot's Guide to Triathlon Training* and to my excitement they outlined a twelve-week training program. Morning after morning of running, biking, or swimming when the rest of the world was still asleep both exhausted and invigorated me. My body soon needed more than nine hours of sleep a night and I ached during my more difficult weeks. During vacations, while my family rested between activities, I was running or swimming. But soon I loved feeling strong as I trimmed seconds off my best times and as difficult, almost impossible things, became easy.

So I had felt confident when I ran into the water for my first triathlon. That feeling disappeared instantly, and I was certain of two things—one, the triathlon was a huge mistake, and two, I hadn't been nearly terrified enough.

With ten family members watching and all that money and time invested, I decided I couldn't quit 5 minutes into the race. In a final attempt to keep going, I started backstroking. It was the only way to breathe. Once I adjusted, I was able to alternate the breaststroke and the backstroke. It was chaos in the water. Several of the other racers were also backstroking, and they would start going sideways and even backwards. One woman wrapped her arm around my neck while she was doing the breaststroke and I had to push her off me. I was grateful when my feet touched the moss-encrusted boat ramp.

I walked up the ramp. I know I should have run but I was glad to be walking. I swallowed so much water from the lake that I was about five miles into the bike ride before I stopped belching.

The bike part was blessedly uneventful. However, if I'm stupid enough to do this again, I'm getting a road bike. Everyone passed me, my only consolation was that I had beaten those same people in the swim.

During the run I made several attempts to drink water but I just spat it out. Any attempt to swallow would have resulted in vomiting. Whose idiotic idea was it to put a steep, rocky hill in the middle of a run? I had nothing left; the desire to turn around and end this was powerful. Up ahead I could see the turnaround point and I knew that no one would know if I turned early. I kept going and made myself physically touch the turnaround chair. One and a half more miles and I was done.

I crossed the finish line and didn't throw up. The pain kept me from feeling joy for a few hours but in the days and months following, I often thought back to that moment and I didn't regret a second. People kept asking if I was going to compete again. I told them maybe.

By the next summer, I had signed up for two more triathlons.

~Melissa Dymock

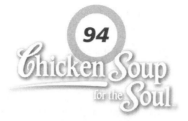

94

Racing with Heart

The most important thing in illness is never to lose heart.
~Nikolai Lenin

"I just want you to know where the AED is in case anything happens to me." My mom pointed out the box on the wall.

I rolled my eyes. I did not think that Mom would need CPR or an AED during the triathlon.

At fifty-seven, my mom would be participating in her first triathlon. I would be competing in my third.

I must have made it look fun the first time she had come and cheered me on, because ever since then she had been talking about signing up for one herself. She signed up for an indoor triathlon at my gym.

We talked over the phone as we prepared for the event. We would both be participating in the mini distance. I was very excited to be in the same race with my mom.

We started our training while still on a waiting list. We were not even sure there would be spots for us in the race but we trained anyway. Two weeks before the race we each got a phone call letting us know that there would be spots open for us. We would be in the same heat.

My mom has always been an inspiration to me for fitness. She made fitness a part of her life and tried to pass that on to us. Every year we got a family gym membership. My sister and I were active on the swim team and my mom swam laps or ran while we practiced.

When my mom took up running we went to races with her and

cheered her on and ran in the kids run. I was excited to compete in an event with her.

When I went home to visit we trained together at her gym.

"I'm so proud of you," she told me while we were swimming laps.

My mom is a strong swimmer. She was concerned about the stationary bike portion and she decided to walk because she had not run in a long time.

On race day she felt ready but nervous.

"I don't want you to wait for me. That makes me nervous because then I feel like I have to keep up with you," Mom said. "Just do your race and I will see you at the finish line."

I finished before my mom and was able to watch her cross the finish line. She had a big smile on her face and she had even run some of her laps around the track.

I was so proud of my mom for participating in the event. I was proud of both of us.

At the end of the race we cooled down and waited for our results to come in.

The next day my mom left to drive back to her home six hours away and I went to work. Later that day I got a phone call from my mom. "I'm in the hospital. I had a heart attack. I don't want you to be worried about me."

Driving home the day after the event my mom felt nauseous and decided to pull over at a hospital. Her work as a cardiac nurse gave her the knowledge that her symptoms might be more than just a stomach flu.

I was shocked. I didn't understand how this had happened. My mom is a fit person. She eats healthy and exercises. She doesn't smoke or drink. She had just completed a triathlon yet here she was in a hospital with a heart attack.

"The doctor said that this was not caused by the triathlon," my sister called later to assure me. It gave me some comfort to know that the event that I had encouraged my mom to sign up for was not the cause of her heart attack.

She spent the next week in the hospital recovering and learning what had caused her heart attack. What she learned is that her heart disease is hereditary. She has low HDLs, which is the good cholesterol. This meant that even though her overall cholesterol number looked okay, the LDLs were high because the HDLs were low. This is a condition that she has even though she exercises and eats right and does all the things that she is supposed to do.

"I guess my triathlon career is on hold for now," she said.

My mom took her time recovering and used her experience to educate her kids about their risks. Exercise was important in her recovery but she had to take it slow at first.

She made sure that we knew that this was hereditary and that we would need to keep an eye on our numbers. She makes sure that we know the importance of exercise and eating right.

I have been able to educate myself and know that heart disease is the number one killer of women. I participate in races that raise money for this cause.

I continue to race in triathlons and running races. It is more important than ever for me to lead a healthy lifestyle.

As for Mom's triathlon career, it isn't over. My mom was back participating in triathlons within a year. She found an event called the Lazyman Triathlon at her gym. Over the course of six weeks my mom swims, bikes and walks the distance of an Ironman triathlon.

~Carrie Monroe

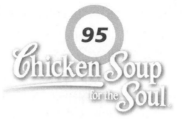

95

In It to Finish

If you set a goal for yourself and are able to achieve it, you have won your
race. Your goal can be to come in first, to improve your performance, or just
finish the race; it's up to you.
~Dave Scott, triathlete

"**W**hy in the world would you drive all that way when you know you aren't even going to finish the race?"

"Thanks for the pep talk, Mom."

Historically, my parents have supported me in whatever I decided to try. But as I was about to get into my car and drive from Wisconsin to Florida to compete in an Ironman triathlon, they thought I was a little crazy. To be fair, my nickname had been "Chunk" while I was in high school. I had always lived by the philosophy that I wasn't going to run unless I was being chased. So with just a couple months of training, maybe it was a bit of a stretch to think that I could swim 2.4 miles, bike 112 miles and run 26.2 miles. Any one of these things by itself would be an incredible feat. Put them all together and it seemed impossible.

I had done my first triathlon a couple of months earlier. It was completely on a whim. I borrowed a bike from a friend of mine and just decided to go for it. Three hours later, I crossed the finish line. The feeling of accomplishment was something that I could never have imagined. It didn't matter that I was one of the last people to finish. I finished.

As soon as it was over, I started looking for more races. I had read about an Ironman distance triathlon that took place in Florida. This wasn't like the one in Hawaii where you had to be an elite athlete to even get to the starting line. For this one, you just paid your entry fee. To make sure people weren't out there for a week, there were cut-off times. You needed to be out of the water by 2 hours 20 minutes. You needed to be off your bike by 10 hours and 30 minutes. And you needed to complete the run by 17 hours. If you didn't hit one of the cutoffs, your race was over. But, if you kept hitting the cutoffs, they let you keep going. That was my plan. Hit the cutoff times and finish. I wasn't out there to win. I was just in it to finish. That was what I kept telling myself: In it to finish.

It was a long drive down to Florida. I kept thinking about what my mom had said. What if I really did drive all that way and didn't finish? What if I didn't make it out of the water in time, and I had to get back in my car for the long drive home, defeated. All of the people that I told about the race would be sure to ask me about it when I got home. How could I tell them that I didn't finish? That would stink, to say the least.

When I finally made it to the race site the night before, I was totally intimidated. There were a few hundred really fit people walking around, and me. This was crazy. I didn't belong here. What was I doing?

I got to my hotel and started getting all of my stuff ready for the next day. I put the race number on my shirt. I put some new laces into my running shoes. Made sure that I had everything ready to go. At the longer races, they have what is called a transition bag. It holds your clothes, and you can put some food in it to help keep you going. I wasn't into all of the special, technical foods like carbohydrate gels or power bars. I made a couple of PB&J sandwiches. I packed a big bag of Chips Ahoy cookies. I figured that I could get through any-thing knowing that I had some cookies waiting for me.

There wasn't a whole lot of sleeping that night. I really just kept thinking about the swim. As long as I made it out of the water in time, I was pretty confident I could finish the race.

The funny thing about an Ironman is that they start everybody at the same time—7 AM. So you have a few hundred people all standing on the edge of the water waiting for the gun to go off. What happens after that can only be described as a human washing machine. Arms and legs flailing around. You get kicked in the face, people trying to swim over you. The group starts to thin out after a while, but the start has all of those people all trying to get to the first buoy at the same time. That's the way it is for everyone—except me. I knew that swimming was not one of my strengths. So rather than dealing with all of that commotion, I just stood on the beach until every other person was in the water and on their way. Then I casually walked in and started my day. I made it around the first lap in just over an hour. For comparison, the fast people were done with the whole 2.4 mile swim before I made it through the first lap. I didn't care. I still had plenty of time to get around before the cutoff. I used every swimming stroke in the book to get my body around that course. Side stroke, back stroke, breast stroke, whatever it took. Two hours and 10 minutes later, I was out of the water. I think I was the last one by about 30 minutes, but all I cared about was that I still had 10 minutes left before the cutoff. Whew.

I was so excited to get on my bike. I had gotten past the swim that could have ended my day early. My excitement didn't last too long as I got my first flat tire right around the 10-mile mark. Fortunately I carried two spare tubes, because I ended up with another flat tire at around 95 miles. I kept on riding, and rolled into the transition area at 5:20 PM. It didn't matter because I had a whole 10 minutes to spare.

I had a strategy. I figured if I could walk really fast, each mile would be around 14 minutes. That would put me into the finish line a little before midnight, and I would be done before the final cutoff of 17 hours. So that is exactly what I did. I never actually ran a step of the 26.2 miles. I walked fast and clicked off each mile on my stopwatch. I crossed the finish line at 16 hours, 40 minutes and 20 seconds on the race clock. I finished. I was now an Ironman.

The next morning I headed back to the race site to pick up my bike and they had pictures that were taken throughout the day, including a photo of me crossing the finish line. The whole ride back to Wisconsin I had the pictures sitting on the passenger seat for me to look at. To remind myself of the fact that I had done it.

That race ended up changing my whole life. I went to graduate school for Sports Administration so I could put on events like that and let other people achieve goals that they might never have thought possible. That is how I met my wife. Together we produced a series of races called the "In It To Finish" duathlon series. We have since completed four Ironman races and over a dozen marathons together. Never looking to win, but always "In It To Finish."

~Chuck Matsoff

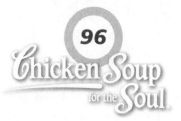

Saying Boo to Cancer

When you think about it, what other choice is there but to hope? We have two
options, medically and emotionally: give up or fight like hell.
~Lance Armstrong

Boo. To me, it's not just a word used to scare ambitious trick-or-treaters on chilling Halloween nights. It's not a decorative term painted on fall home furnishings either. Surprisingly, it is the unique name of my mom—a Sylvania, Ohio, resident lovingly known by her family and close friends as "The Lance Armstrong of Ohio." Boo Hensien did not compete in the Tour de France but she did snag the third place trophy in the Sylvania Triathlon. Doesn't sound too impressive? Well she did it two days after she completed her last radiation treatment in her fight against breast cancer.

It was a snowy February day when my mom found a lump in her left breast. She didn't tell me. It was just a few days before my twelfth birthday and she didn't want to ruin my excitement. The very next day the lump was biopsied. Two days later was a day my mom will never forget, in fact it is a day that she remembers in extreme detail. She was seated Indian style on the kelly green carpet of her bedroom floor, folding my father's white v-neck undershirt when the telephone rang. It was one word from the voice on the other side of line that made her heart drop. One word that made her body drop back down to the carpet she had been sitting on just seconds earlier. One word that made that cold February day the scariest of her life. Cancer.

Staying true to character, it only took my mom a few hours, and some comforting from her best friend Karen, to design a foolproof plan to defeat this sudden opponent. Step one was educating herself. She researched, read, consulted specialists and took plenty of notes in order to choose the best treatment plan for her condition. She ended up deciding on a lumpectomy and chemo and radiation therapy. She also decided that she "wanted to see what the body was capable of when placed in a really stressful situation." So, as soon as she implemented her plan for recovery she also executed her training plan for the Sylvania Triathlon.

As soon as chemo and radiation treatments began so did my mother's training for the big race. I specifically remember grade school mornings when my mom would make me eggs, then lean over the toilet bowl emptying herself of last night's dinner, then immediately lace up her running shoes for that morning's workout. Her training consisted of 10- to 12-mile runs, five days a week, as well as two days of swimming at least a mile or more—all of this completed while battling the fatigue and nausea brought on by her chemotherapy.

Everything about my mother's battle was positive. In fact, I don't even remember ever feeling a hint of nervousness or apprehension about her diagnosis. I don't think I ever even thought of cancer as a life-threatening disease. My mom treated it as if it were a common cold, nothing that would affect or slow down her normal daily activities.

My favorite memory of the whole process occurred right before my mom's chemo treatments began. It was a typical school day in my seventh-grade world until I was called down to the principal's office. I was told that I was being picked up to go home, possibly the best news a twelve-year-old could ever receive! When I arrived at my house, my haircutter of eleven years, Kevin Charles, was there with his shears, electric razor and a huge smile. We strapped down my giggling mother with a plastic drape to catch the massive amounts of hair that would soon be falling from her head. We then pulled her wiry strawberry-blond locks into a long braid which was fastened securely on top of her head. Kevin prepared me for my first haircutting experience by instructing me on how to use an electric razor.

Just minutes later my mom was left with just the braid, the rest of her head bald. After taking many Polaroids of the bald babe with the braid, the long-lasting lock was easily snipped off leaving my mother's head completely hairless. She looked in her hand mirror and said, "I even look beautiful bald."

Five months and hundreds of miles later it was time for my mom's thirty-third and final radiation treatment. Two days after that it was time for the Sylvania Triathlon. Donning a two-piece Speedo swimsuit and a yellow ball cap, my mom was ready to compete. What happened next not only shocked my family, friends and the newspaper writers and photographers who had gathered for the amazing race, but even astounded the four oncologists who had been treating my mom. My forty-five-year-old mom not only finished the triathlon, but she did it in 2:38:12, only 13 minutes slower than her best-ever time, which was achieved when she was thirty-eight years old and cancer-free. She also placed third out of all the women who were competing in her age group.

Boo Hensien is a cancer survivor and a triathlete, but more importantly she is my mom. I have watched her struggle, I have watched her succeed, and through all of it I have watched her continue to be the best mom I could have ever asked for. I am twenty-one years old now. It has been nine years since my mom's battle with breast cancer. Not once in those nine years has my admiration and amazement towards my mother faded, and I'm pretty sure it never will.

~Molly Hensien

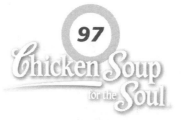

97

Twenty Years to Reach a Pipe Dream

You can't put a limit on anything. The more you dream, the farther you get.
~Michael Phelps

"But I'm not a runner," I said.

"It doesn't matter. You can walk part, run part. That's what we did last year," said the woman next to me as we toweled off in the locker room after swim practice.

I was in awe of my teammates—middle-aged women like me—who were talking about participating in an upcoming sprint triathlon. Competing in a triathlon had been my pipe dream for twenty years, ever since I had watched an in-flight movie about the Ironman Triathlon on my way to Hawaii. The fantasy was an ocean away from the reality of my Midwestern life.

I wasn't a swimmer, biker, or runner. At that time my only exercise was chasing after my three little boys. I loved being with my kids. Taking time away from them to train wasn't even a consideration. I had grown up in a time and place where girls' athletics were almost non-existent. It wasn't a matter of getting back into shape. I didn't have a clue where to begin.

When the boys got older I bought a bike and discovered that I loved the adrenaline buzz from the exercise. Biking was easy. I wasn't fast, but I had endurance and relished biking long distances.

A few years ago I went on a bike trip in the Canadian Rockies with four other women. When my friend in New York told her colleagues about the trip, they told her she wouldn't be able to do it. "How hard can it be? I'm going with four middle-aged women from Chicago," she said.

The rest of us repeated "how hard can it be?" to her as we labored up the mountains. Although I found it necessary to "stop to admire the view" occasionally on the uphill climbs, I had the satisfaction of completing the entire route. I was a biker—but I still didn't swim or run.

Not knowing that I wasn't a swimmer, a friend invited me to join her at her swim team practice a couple of years ago. I trusted her when she said that the team was for adults at all ability levels. My body ached when I got into bed after that first practice. The coaches' instructions and the other swimmers' encouragement convinced me to join the team. As my middle-aged body worked muscles I hadn't known existed, I discovered the exhilaration of a tough swim work-out. I was starting from nothing so all I could do was improve.

The team expected everyone to compete in the state meet. I had a conflict the first year, but I didn't have any excuse the second. Although I was one of the slowest swimmers on our team, I had endurance. I had trouble keeping track of distance and time so one of my coaches wrote my registration information on a scrap of paper for me. My biggest fear when I signed up online was that I would make a mistake and put down a time that was faster than Michael Phelps.

I had never even seen a swim meet before. I was afraid I'd show up at the wrong place and miss my races, my goggles would slip off, and I'd lose track of how many laps to swim. I met my goals—I signed up, showed up, and swam. The icing on the cake was winning four ribbons. I was a swimmer—but I still didn't run.

The ladies in the locker room had given me the key to being a triathlete. I didn't have to run—I could walk. The next day I bought my first pair of running shoes and a bike rack for my car and reg-istered for my first triathlon. It was my oldest child's twenty-eighth birthday.

Four days later, with "381" written on my arms and legs and a timing chip around my ankle, I jumped into the water. The 300-

meter swim was shorter than my team's usual warm up. It almost didn't seem worth getting wet for.

The 10-mile bike ride on traffic-free, smooth streets with cheering onlookers was a breeze. As I left the bike corral, I jogged. I couldn't pace myself because I didn't have any concept of my speed, time, or distance. I got past the cheering throng before I started walking.

When a seventyish man slowly jogged past me, I decided to use him to set my pace. I started running again. Volunteers along the route handed out water bottles as we ran by. He took one. I took one. He poured the water over his head. I poured the water over my head. He tossed his empty bottle on the ground. I held onto mine as I ran and looked for a recycling bin. I didn't know the protocol. Littering didn't seem right. Then I noticed lots of bottles on the ground and realized that volunteers would be picking them up. Runners were supposed to be concentrating on running, not on recycling. I tossed my empty bottle on the ground.

The man kept running and I couldn't keep up. My pace slowed and I started walking again. I alternated running and walking. A spectator cheered "You are almost there!" I picked up my pace and thought "I can do this! I'm going to run across the finish line." I rounded the next bend expecting to be steps from my destination. I wasn't, but I was close enough to the cheering crowd that I was too embarrassed to start walking again. I pushed myself and ran across the finish line. Seconds later someone slipped a medal on a ribbon over my head.

Of the 400 people who had entered the competition, 363 completed it. I was older than 340 of them.

I'm still not a runner, but after twenty years my pipe dream is a reality. The triangular medal pinned on my bulletin board reminds me—I'm a triathlete.

~Karen Gray-Keeler

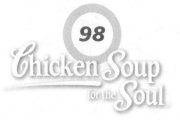

98

The Heart of an Ironman

A winner's strongest muscle is her heart.
~Cassie Campbell

Surely the driver could see me.

A split second later, I went for the brakes. But it was too late and as the front wheel of my bicycle hit the bumper of her car, I was thrown into the windshield.

Rolling off the car and lying on the ground, I felt as though my body had become disconnected. My legs floated in mid-air. I couldn't feel anything below my waist. I struggled for every breath. A few hours and many medical tests later, doctors confirmed a T-4 (chest level) spinal cord injury.

I would never walk again.

Earlier that morning, I'd stood in front of the mirror, staring at my five foot, eleven inch frame. I was in the best shape of my life. My long legs were lean, yet muscular, suggesting that I had logged many hours in the gym and on the bicycle. Having just completed my final races of the season, I was on top of the world. I knew it was time to turn it down a notch and take it easy. Still, my friend Matt and I headed to Lookout Mountain, just to feel the breeze on our faces and enjoy the sunny fall day. It began like any other ride, but by the end of the day in the Intensive Care Unit, my life took a turn down a whole new path.

As I lay four months in the rehabilitation hospital, as a bike racer who now had no use of her legs, I knew that in my case, the word "former" would always precede the word "cyclist."

In a moment, I had gone from being an independent athlete who had spent two months alone, traveling the country and competing in races, to having to re-learn the most basic of life skills—getting in and out of bed, opening doors and learning to drive with my hands.

Five years and thousands of hours of physical therapy, rehabilitation and intense physical training later, I sat under the moon on the shore of Lake Hefner, in Oklahoma City, pulling a wetsuit onto my unresponsive legs. With every tug of the neoprene, my thoughts turned to the seemingly insurmountable task in front of me. What was I thinking? Could I really do this? Could I complete a 2.4-mile swim, then a 112-mile bike ride (on a handcycle), followed by a 26.2-mile run (in a racing chair), all in 17 hours?

When I told my coach, Neal, that I wanted to attempt an Ironman, he didn't flinch at the idea. When I saw the training program he designed for me, I nearly fell out of my wheelchair. I had visions of what I would look like if my arms just fell off.

So there I was, entered in the Redman race in Oklahoma, preparing to make a mark in wheelchair racing history. Since I would be the only wheelchair racer among a field of 3,000 participants, I'd be in constant contact with the race director, Roger, so he could assist with my accessibility and race equipment.

At the race meeting, my boyfriend Steve and I listened as Roger announced that there were many first-timers registered for the event. He would not enforce the 17-hour cutoff for anyone. "If you're still out there and you're going to come in at 21 hours, I will be there at the finish line waiting for you." That was a big relief. Now it was up to me and my physical conditioning as to whether I would cross the finish line or not.

At that meeting, I met the only other disabled participant, John, a below-the-knee amputee. "We're going to get through this race!" he cheered.

Now, at 7:00 AM, Neal stood next to me as I sat in the water. Because of my injury, it was easier to swim backstroke so I had him as a guide swimmer to direct me through the water. Neal would yell, "Left," "Right," or point directly over my line of sight so I could stay on course, though I could barely see him through my dark goggles.

When the mass swim began, I swam over swimmers, unable to find a good space in the pack. But I kept up and even passed quite a few people. Finally I concentrated on Neal's directions, and settled in for the long ride. I swam with my head up just a bit to see his hand signals, my neck muscles aching fiercely. I put my head back often, with my face totally underwater, and hoped and prayed I could keep an eye on Neal.

We hit shore at 1 hour 45 minutes and Steve and Roger rushed in, picked me up and rushed me to my wheelchair. My team gathered around me and took off my wetsuit. I was pushed into the changing tent, lightheaded and foggy. Two women threw my cycling jersey on me, handed me food and drink, got me in my handcycle, and I was off.

The first part of the 28-mile loop was flat, but it soon became hilly. One male racer passed me and said, "You're awesome and you're beautiful!" I smiled and kept pushing. As I was closing in on the end of the first loop, my average speed was dropping quickly and I began to get discouraged. I still had three laps to go.

When I got to transition, Steve and Neal were waiting for me, so I smiled as I passed and tried to get psyched for a second lap. But I was starting to feel sick. My stomach hurt from all the energy bars, gels and drink I'd ingested. The temperature was rising into the 90s.

As I pulled into transition the second time, I wondered if it was time to call the race. I felt like throwing up and expected to collapse at any moment. "Maybe I should quit," I gasped to Neal and Steve. "It's past 3:00 and two more laps will take at least six hours… it'll be past 9:00 by the time I start the run."

Neal said, "Well, you still have sunlight." I gathered that meant stop whining and keep going. It's hard to get sympathy from an accomplished distance athlete as your coach.

"Keep the van close to me," I said as I headed out again. Steve got on his bike to ride with me to make sure I was safe. As we rode I went back and forth between whining and crying, wanting to give up. Steve turned to me. "If it's your body that's telling you to quit, go ahead, but if it's your mind, you need to keep going, otherwise you'll regret it."

He was right. I didn't come this far to be a quitter.

When we arrived in transition at the end of the third lap, Roger was there. "Are you sure you want to keep going?" he asked. Everyone else was off the course and the road was opening to traffic.

I can have doubts about my abilities, but I refuse to have others doubt me.

"I'll be fine!" Then to Steve and Neal, "Let's go!"

Neal painted "Race Support" on the back window of the van and followed Steve and me closely as we rode into the sunset. The air got cooler, the sky darker. My stomach was so inflamed, it was hard to eat or drink.

As we approached the final turn Steve encouraged, "You're home free now!"

I thought to myself, "You know you've had a long day when 'only' having to finish a marathon is a relief!"

The transition area looked like a ghost town when I pulled in. All of the other racers were either already on the running course or had finished and were at home sleeping in bed.

With shaking arms, I quickly transferred from my handcycle to my racing chair to do the "run." Steve continued on his bike and led me through the dark winding path. Exhausted, we rode in silence. As we hit the turnaround, one of the volunteers told us we were on pace to finish in three hours. "You have got to be kidding!" I thought. "THREE hours? I have been going since 7 AM!"

On we pushed.

Many miles and hours later, we saw big spotlights ahead. Steve pulled off the path and said, "It's all yours!"

I pushed as hard as I could to the finish. There wasn't an overwhelming crowd waiting for me as I had played over and over in my mind. Instead there were only a handful of volunteers as I crossed the line at 1:03 AM, 18 hours and 3 minutes after I had begun.

And there, true to his word, was Roger, waiting to put the Ironman finisher's medal around my neck.

I thought I might doubt my status as an Ironman, having missed the 17-hour cutoff mark. I realized then that nothing in life is only about hours and minutes—it's about heart.

Right then and there, I knew I had the heart of an Ironman.

~Tricia Downing

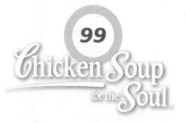

99

Racing Back

What you fear is that which requires action to overcome.
~Byron Pulsifer

"I'm going to sign up for the triathlon," Tammy said over coffee.

"The Splash, Pedal and Gasp?" I put my mug down and stared at her, "The one on Mother's Day?"

"That's the one. I'm going to sign up with you and Heather."

"But you don't know how to swim."

Tammy shrugged, "Well, I guess I better learn."

Tammy, Heather and I had been working out together for a few years, and needing a bigger challenge for our workouts, we'd recently set the goal of completing individual triathlons. The only problem with this plan was Tammy didn't know how to swim. Before she was born, her uncle had died in a tragic drowning accident and her mother wouldn't let her near the water. Now as an adult Tammy faced the daunting task of overcoming her own fear of water.

Our friend Todd happened to be the coach for the masters swim club in town, and with a little prodding, we signed up for coaching sessions. Twice a week, while Todd corrected my stroke, and I splashed my way down the length of the pool trying to whip myself into shape, Tammy would be in the lane next to me, quietly struggling with the basics that I took for granted.

With a float around her waist, Tammy slowly learned to put her face underwater, blowing bubbles without panicking. Eventually, the float was gone, and Tammy was working her way down the lane. Todd celebrated every small achievement by calling over to me, "Elena, look. She's kicking." Or, "Elena, she's not using fins."

In a few short weeks, Todd had her working on her backstroke, until one night he stopped me at the end of my lane bursting with pride, "Elena, check it out! She's swimming, she's swimming."

I hopped onto the pool deck to watch Tammy swim the length of the pool on her back. Later, in the hot tub, we celebrated her success.

"Tammy, that's awesome. You were swimming!"

"Yeah, on my back."

"Who cares if it was on your back?"

"It's backstroke. I need to learn front stroke."

"Tammy, you were swimming. That's huge."

"Thanks, Elena. But I can't swim a race on my back."

I looked her in the eyes and said, "Why not?"

For the next few weeks, the three of us would run and cycle together, training for the upcoming race. But Monday and Wednesday nights would find us back in the pool. Tammy painstakingly worked on the basics of the crawl. With every stroke she took, she fought her fears and confronted her nemesis.

Finally, the weekend of the race was upon us. We loaded up our gear and our families and made the trip two hours south to the University of Lethbridge, my alma mater. We left the husbands in charge of the children at the hotel and Heather, Tammy and I went to check out the venue and pick up our race packages.

Excitement filled the air as I checked out all the changes to the school I hadn't been to in almost a decade. Heather pointed out the similarities in the Olympic length pool to those she used to race in. Only Tammy was suspiciously quiet. She sat in the risers, looking over the pool, studying it. Taking in the cool blue of the water, the colorful lane markers, but most importantly, the 25-meter length difference from the pool at home that we'd trained in. She didn't say much for the rest of the night, retreating into her private world of reflection.

On race day, the stands were full of spectators, our families included. We watched in anticipation as the athletes racing in the Olympic and sprint length triathlons started. We were registered for the shorter, introductory distance of a super-sprint. Finally, it was our turn. We hugged each other before jumping into the pool in our assigned lanes to warm up and take our marks. From my spot in the water, I looked over at Tammy still on the pool deck and silently willed her to get in the water, not to back out, not to give in to her fears. She got in.

After the whistle blew, I didn't see Tammy again until after the turn around on the bike portion of the race. When I saw her light blue jersey, I cheered and called out, the sting of tears coming to my eyes because I knew she'd done it. She swam.

Our finishing times didn't matter. As we each came across the finish line to hugs and cheers from our husbands and children, we all knew what mattered that day. Over a celebratory lunch, we recapped the events and learned that Tammy's swim hadn't gone as smoothly as we'd hoped. In the flurry of swimmers, arms and legs flailing, she'd experienced a moment of panic. A moment where she considered quitting, pulling herself out of the pool and not finishing the race. She didn't. She flipped to her back and completed the race doing backstroke. All three of us accomplished a physical challenge, but my best friend taught me a valuable lesson that day. No matter what your fears are, if you can dream it—you can do it. And as it turns out, you can do backstroke in a race!

~Elena Aitken

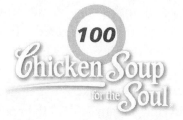

Competing Voices

One advantage of talking to yourself is that you know at least somebody's listening.
~Franklin P. Jones

I have a voice in my head. No, I'm not crazy, but I do have this voice that worries about things like missing Visa bills and whether or not I should let my five-year-old anywhere near the rock wall at school. When I exercise the voice tends to whine. *Your ankle hurts. Other people aren't breathing this hard. You have no coordination whatsoever.* Things like that. However, one afternoon as I was chit-chatting with another mom and she began telling me about the triathlon she'd just completed, something unusual happened.

The voice in my head said, *Oh yeah, you're going to kick ass.*

Now, this was new. My voice was normally much more Woody Allen than Sylvester Stallone. It did not make presumptions about my physical abilities. I ran a little, mostly on a treadmill at the gym, but even on my best days I was a slow and reluctant runner. A Vespa in highway traffic. Really I'm not really a runner at all.

Nevertheless, that winter my friend and I signed up for the Danskin Women's Triathlon New York Metro race, which was a half-mile swim, an 11-mile bike ride, and a 5K run. We had until September to prepare.

I can swim but have never been a particularly strong swimmer, so I decided that an intermediate swim class would be a good place to start. That first week a single lap of crawl stroke left me breathless and exhausted. My instructor started me on some drills.

You have six months, my voice said. *No worries.* On the other hand, face in the pool, the worrier in me was in full force. Mostly, she whined. *This sucks. You are a terrible swimmer. You can only breathe on one side and you're completely wrecked after two laps. This is very, very bad.*

When spring arrived, I started running a 2.8 mile loop through the local neighborhoods around the gym. I was slow, but I could run the whole thing without stopping. In May I ran a 5K race.

See? I thought. *You can do this. No problem.*

However, I was dodging the bike situation. My husband had a hybrid bike, but I was afraid to actually ride it any distance because I was positive that flat tires, thrown chains, and various other mechanical misfortunes would leave me stranded on the side of the road somewhere.

My stepfather, however, decided I needed a bike of my own. He found me a road bike on eBay.

"Now you have to perform," he said.

Uh oh.

My first ride on the new bike was not particularly successful. I could not figure out how to change the gears. It was in a very low gear and I rode all around the neighborhood spinning like mad, trying to figure out how to make the gears go higher. There didn't seem to be anything to adjust. *Maybe it's broken,* I thought. *Maybe there's a missing part.* Then I thought, *maybe you're a forty-year-old woman who can't figure out how to shift a freaking bicycle.*

As I headed for home, pedals spinning wildly, I felt my imminent humiliation. I gave it one last effort, tinkering with anything and everything, and realized there were little tabs hidden under the brakes. Everything shifted to the side, making the gears go higher and lower.

Oh thank God.

I swam, biked and ran as often as I could, building up to 20-mile bike rides and 5-mile runs. Swimming was still my weakest area, but I was able to comfortably swim forty laps in the pool. Ideally I knew I needed to practice in open water, but the circumstances for that never quite came together.

Not to worry, you've come a long way. You can only do so much.

Triathlon day arrived. I was nervous, obviously. *You're not going to be able to swim that far, you will never manage to change a tire if you get a flat, and your knees don't really feel up to this* were some of my most frequent concerns. However, I was also excited about finally making it to the big day. *You did great. You're ready.*

By the time I was waiting for my swim wave I was so nervous I was jumping in place.

"Cold?" my friend asked.

"No, I've got my panic to keep me warm," I joked, except I wasn't joking. I was truly starting to freak out.

There were so many bodies and colored caps on the beach in front of me I couldn't see the water. I waited for the announcer to call my wave. I was the 13th wave, in yellow caps. *Unluckiest number and the color of cowards. Fabulous.* When my wave was called, I waded into the water.

"Go!"

As soon as I put my face in the water it was obvious that I was in trouble. It was like I was in a blender. *OH MY GOD!* Everything was in motion, churning brown and white and body parts. I started doing the crawl but when I turned my head to breathe I got smacked in the face by the choppy water. I couldn't see anything. I managed a few strokes but my heart was racing and I was already out of breath. I struggled for any forward motion. The buoys that had looked fairly reasonable from the beach looked very, very far away. My goggles were fogging. Everything was going wrong.

I started treading water and noticed that the other yellow caps were starting to pull away. All of a sudden the voice in my head changed. *If you let your wave get away you're done! DO NOT LOSE YOUR WAVE!* Like the flipping of a switch my focus changed from being about swim strokes and murky, choppy water, to being about the wave. I had to keep up. I crawled, breaststroked, sidestroked, doggie paddled, and just plain grappled my way along, determined to keep the yellow caps around me. One by one the buoys passed. Soon, I could see the finish.

Putting my feet back in the sand was pure euphoria. Far from being exhausted by my manic effort, I had never felt lighter than I did as I ran up the beach, officially ending my swim.

The bike and the run went well. On the bike, my mind remained calm and focused on logistics. *Drink water. Have a GU. Don't overdo it.* I had a good, fast ride.

The run was a little rough at first with my wobbly bike legs but I saw my family cheering me on and reminded myself, *this is the easy part. It's as simple as one foot in front of the other.* I found a comfortable pace and the miles passed. As I crossed the finish line, I don't think I have ever felt so strong, so proud in my whole life.

At the end, my mind was empty. If it is possible for a brain to simply smile, that's what mine did. I had done it, and done it well, finishing in 1:21:44, better than the hour and a half I had been hoping for.

I can't wait to do it again!

~Christina Kapp

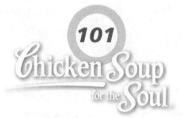

Triathlete Grandma

When anyone tells me I can't do anything... I'm just not listening any more.
~Florence Griffith Joyner

When I run a 5K, I usually ask myself why I am doing this before the end of the first mile. Most runners have passed me, I feel the blood rushing to my cheeks, and my breathing is labored. Nevertheless, with sheer determination and a steady pace, this grandma keeps moving forward.

Near the end of the second mile I begin to relax. Becoming a runner at forty-eight taught me that no one can run my race for me. To reach the finish line, I must run according to my abilities, not others'. Once I've passed the halfway point, I press on under the illusion of saving myself for a big finish. The finish is rarely big, but I always finish.

The challenges at my age go beyond physical. Training for a race also challenges me mentally and emotionally, and parallels how I live life. At the start of a race, the distance between the beginning and the end is daunting. To finish I focus on where I am rather than where I'm going. The same is true of my daily challenges. When I set goals and move toward them one step at a time, the journey doesn't seem so overwhelming and I get to enjoy the scenery along the way.

Becoming athletic at my age is also a way to keep a handle on my cholesterol levels, blood pressure, and a slew of other physical maladies that creep into a senior's life. In the greater race of life, I want to cross the final finish line strong, knowing that I persevered in the challenges of the race, kept going when I didn't believe I could take another step, and smiled victoriously at those who cheered me on.

My family surprised me with a road bike for my fiftieth birthday. I thought it was the coolest gift ever for a grandmother of six and immediately joined a bicycle club. We rode every weekend during the summer, riding anywhere from fifty to eighty miles a day. On one occasion, we pedaled a hundred miles over the country roads of Illinois.

At the age of fifty-two, I was diagnosed with breast cancer. The surgery and radiation treatments left my muscles so tender that I couldn't lift my left arm above my head without pain. Already uncomfortable with arthritis in my neck, feet and hands, I decided to wage a battle against the pain and join the YMCA.

My first time in the pool found me huffing, puffing, and gasping for air at the end of the first lap. While stubbornness had not always served me well, in this instance it did. Soon I was swimming three times a week and, in time, joined the Masters Swim Team. Skepticism was apparent on my instructor's face, a young man who was far more at ease training ironman triathletes and marathon runners than a senior citizen. Although I was out of my league in athletic ability, no one could question my determination to persevere in the drills and laps.

As I became more experienced, I ran several 5K and 8K races with my boss, a forty-year-old woman and long time triathlete. Physical training and endurance were the weapons of choice in her battle with rheumatoid arthritis. We were having lunch one day when she asked, "Bonnie, you bike, run, and swim, so why not sign up for a triathlon?" So, I did.

My goal in my first triathlon was to make it to the finish line. When I placed second in my age group, I was astonished. That there were only two of us in my age group didn't diminish my sense of accomplishment. I figured that being one of only two in my category in a field of 2,000 women was a statement in itself. So with great pride, I hung my medal on a hook in the garage, right next to the rakes, shovels, and other garden tools.

I entered the triathlon the following year and placed second again, but this time there were six in my age group. When the medal was placed around my neck, I shed a triumphant tear and felt like a real champion.

In the world of athletics I'm the tortoise, not the hare. Even so, I find great rewards in pushing myself to my limits. It's me finding out who I really am when alone on the trail with no one to measure my distance but me. It's me finding out my true character when counting my laps and no one else is around. It's me not giving up when exhausted and continuing to grind my way to the end. I have the wonderful sense of accomplishment that comes with victory over physical and mental challenges, knowing that I did the best I could with what I have been given.

Because I am sixty-six, my eighty-five-year-old mother worries that I will have a heart attack during a race. My response is always the same: "Mother, I would rather die falling off my bike than falling off the couch."

~Bonnie Schey McClurg

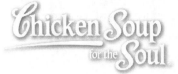

Meet Our Contributors

Elena Aitken lives in Alberta, Canada, where she spends her time hanging out with her seven-year-old twins, training for various athletic events and writing. She's currently looking for a publisher for her first novel. She can be reached at elena@inkblotcommunications. ca or www.inkblotcommunications.ca.

Michelle Barton lives and trains in Orange County, CA. She enjoys running ultramarathons every month and trail races with her dad and daughter. Michelle also enjoys mountain biking, swimming, coaching her daughter's soccer team and choreographing her daughter's talent show. She looks forward to running the Badwater 135-mile Ultramarathon and the 211-mile John Muir Trail.

Jill Barville lives, writes and runs in Spokane, WA, home to Bloomsday, one of the world's largest road races. Her work has appeared in *The Spokesman-Review*, multiple magazines and she is writing her first novel. Contact her via e-mail at jbarville@msn.com.

Tina Bausinger has published several poems, some short stories, and writes a humor column for the University of Texas at Tyler *Patriot Talon*. She is a wife and a mother of three. She is currently working towards her goal of becoming an English teacher, and has finished her first novel. Please e-mail her at tinaboss71@yahoo.com.

R. Mike Bennett is the editorial content manager for the United Church of God. He and his wife have two wonderful daughters, and he shares his thoughts on his blog "Forward to the Kingdom" at http://ucgmikebennett.wordpress.com.

Melissa Blanco is a graduate of Gonzaga University. She lives in Washington with her husband and three children. Please visit her website at www.melissablanco.com.

Charles Boyle worked thirty-five years at NASA. He is the author of *Shuttle Rising: Rendezvous with a Rumor*, and two kids' picture books titled *Tailey Whaley* and *The Sandpiper's Game*. He is a scuba diver and sailor.

Julie Bradford Brand received her BS from Susquehanna University and went on to attend NYU toward her MBA. She worked in human resources before deciding to stay home with her children. Julie enjoys running, writing, and spending time with her family. She also loves being a part of her book club!

Michael Brennan's first race, the Terry Fox half marathon in 1980, was his way of honouring his ailing mother and Terry Fox. It launched a career in running spanning 57 marathons, years of coaching thousands of runners, and now organizing races from 5K to marathon.

Tim Brewster is an outdoor enthusiast in Alberta, Canada. He loves skiing, cycling, hiking, and fishing with his two daughters and wife Cindy. Someday he hopes to turn the tales he made up for his kids into children's books.

Christine A. Brooks is a writer, ocean activist, environmentalist, and surfer who believes in writing about the wonderful path that has led to meeting many wonderful people and learning their stories. She lives with her family and very opinionated dog, Harley. Christine is currently finishing her second book, *A Voice to be Heard*. Contact her at chris@fourleafclover.us.

John P. Buentello is a writer who has published essays, fiction, and poetry. He is the co-author of the novel *Reproduction Rights* and the story collection *Binary Tales*. He is at work on a new novel and a picture book for children. He can be reached via e-mail at jakkhakk@yahoo.com.

Melissa Butler is a self-proclaimed adventurer. She began journaling her life nearly twenty-five years ago and continues today. An avid long distance runner, Melissa enjoys running ultramarathons and looks forward to hiking to Mount Everest base camp. She is an artist, animal lover and lives a minimalistic lifestyle. E-mail her at missmatt@iowatelecom.net.

Cristina Cherry is a resident of Central Illinois. She lives with her husband, two sons, two cats, and a bunny. Cristina enjoys reading, writing, running and hiking. She plans to continue writing inspirational fiction and non-fiction for children and adults. E-mail Cristina at cristinacherry@hotmail.com.

Josh Cox is a writer, speaker, TV personality, and professional marathon runner. Josh, the 50K American Record Holder, is a four-time Olympic Trials Qualifier and three-time US National Team member. His book, *Soul Runners*, co-written with his training partner, Ryan Hall, is due out in 2011. For inquiries: admin@joshcox.com, www.joshcox.com.

Luci L. Creery lives and teaches in Arizona where she is pursuing a Master of Arts degree in English and, more importantly, happily raising five children with her husband, Adam. In her spare time (which there is not much of), she runs to stay in shape, to escape, and to stay sane.

Bob Dickson lives with his wife and two daughters in Southern California. He's written for the *Los Angeles Daily News*, Santa Clarita's *The Signal, the Los Angeles Times* Newspaper Group, and has been published in several books and magazines. He also teaches writing at The Master's College. Bob can be reached at Bob@BobsWordFactory.com.

On September 17, 2000, **Tricia Downing** was hit by a car while riding her bike. Although paralyzed from the chest down, she returned to sports and has completed over fifty triathlons. She is a motivational speaker and holds degrees in Journalism, Sports Management and Disability Studies. Please e-mail her at ladyterp_td@hotmail.com.

Marie Duffoo is a full-time writer and animal activist. When she is not writing she spends her time rescuing sick, abandoned and injured animals.

Christina Dymock graduated from the University of Utah. She currently resides in a small town in Central Utah with her husband and four children. Among other things, she enjoys running, cross country skiing, wakeboarding, sewing, reading and baking. Watch for her children's popcorn cookbook to be released in the spring of 2011.

Melissa Dymock graduated from Utah State with a degree in Journalism. She is a writer and editor and lives in Salt Lake City, Utah. When it's too snowy to train for triathlons, she hits the ski slopes. Please e-mail her at rmrd23@yahoo.com.

James S. Fell, MBA, CSCS, is a husband, father, runner, weightlifter and fitness writer. In addition to writing for a variety of respected fitness magazines, he is the author of *Body for Wife: The Family Guy's Guide to Getting in Shape*. Visit www.bodyforwife.com or e-mail him at james@bodyforwife.com.

Matt Fitzgerald is a senior editor of *Triathlete Magazine* and a senior online producer for RunNow.com. He has written numerous books for triathletes and runners, including *RUN: The Mind-Body Method of Running by Feel*. He lives and runs in San Diego with his wife, Nataki.

Janine Fleury, a veteran of sixteen marathons, including Boston, was raised by her grandmother in the village of Novogrod in communist Poland. At fifteen, Janine fled to America, penniless and speaking no English. Forty years later, Janine returned to her homeland as a journalist for *Running Times* magazine and competed in the Warsaw Marathon.

Jennifer Freed teaches high school English and writing classes. She received an MFA in creative writing from Wilkes University in 2008. She lives in Lewistown, Pennsylvania with her three children.

Marian Tascio Friedrichs is a freelance writer from New York, where she earned her Master of Arts degree in Writing from Manhattanville College. Marian writes essays, articles, and reviews for several print and online publications. She loves Catholic churches, good coffeehouses, and the smell of old books. Contact her via e-mail at mtascio@yahoo.com.

Jenny R. George lives on a five-acre hobby farm north of Coeur d'Alene, ID with her husband, two children and a menagerie of animals. This is Jenny's second published story for *Chicken Soup for the Soul*. Her first story, "Dusting Off Memories", appeared in *Chicken Soup for the Soul: Thanks Mom*.

Elizabeth Kathryn Gerold-Miller is a write-at-home mother of four residing on Long Island. She writes a blog, "The Divine Gift of Motherhood" and trains her children to run cross country. Please e-mail her at ekgeroldmiller@gmail.com.

Courtney Gilman completed her Peace Corps service in April 2009. She resides in Norman, OK, and manages the non-profit organization, Touchstone Youth Project, in which disadvantaged youth cultivate life skills through the challenging sport of rock climbing. Courtney received her Masters of Social Work in 2006. Contact her at cmgilman@touchstoneyouth.org or http://courtinthegambia.blogspot.com.

Shelby Gonzalez is a nature and science writer with over 100 articles to her credit. Formerly a rock climbing instructor, she runs, climbs, and travels often (four continents and counting!). She is working on her first novel and planning her wedding with her surfer fiancé. Her website is www.ShelbyGonzalez.com.

Karen Gray-Keeler appreciates that her family encourages her pipe dreams. She contributed to *Chicken Soup for the Soul: Empty Nesters* and dreams of completing her first book—but opportunities for new adventures keep beckoning her. Karen and her husband Tom live in the Chicago area and enjoy having their family nearby.

Lee Hammerschmidt is a graphic designer/writer/songwriter/troubadour/Zen master who lives on the fringe of Portland, OR. His work has appeared in multiple publications and websites.

Cindy Hanna is a mother of four who runs races and obstacle courses, is a novelist, freelance writer, and author of her own website, www.cindyhanna.com, where she interacts with her readers. She also publishes and edits her own e-zine, www.InspireME.me, which provides information for a healthy mind, body and soul.

Gil D. Hannon lives in Tinley Park, IL with his amazing wife and three beautiful children. He works as a financial advisor. Gil enjoys triathlon competition along with skiing, sailing, hiking, and outdoor adventures that bring him closer to nature. Feel free to e-mail him at gil4peace@comcast.net.

Dena Harris started running with geezers in December 2006. She has since qualified for and run Boston. An award-winning humor writer, Dena lives in North Carolina with her husband and two cats, all of whom glaze over when she talks—frequently—about running. Visit Dena online at www.denaharris.com.

Lori Hein is the author of *Ribbons of Highway: A Mother-Child Journey Across America*. Her freelance work has appeared in the *Boston Globe* and several *Chicken Soup for the Soul* titles. Visit her at www.LoriHein.com or her world travel blog, www.RibbonsofHighway.blogspot.com.

Molly Hensien received her bachelor's degree in Journalism from the University of Dayton in 2010. She hopes to be training dolphins or working in the Peace Corps by the time this paragraph is read. Molly hopes to eventually attend veterinary school.

Beth Braccio Hering graduated from Northwestern University in 1990 with honors in Sociology. After years of working on *Encyclopædia Britannica* products, she now freelances from her Chicago home. Beth's favorite subjects to write about include parenting, education, celebrities, ice skating, and the Chicago Cubs. Please e-mail her at BBHering@aol.com.

Ginger Herring majored in Creative Writing at Eckerd College. Her poem, "Dad's Backyard," was selected for publication on the Online International Poetry Competition website for VoicesNet. Ginger continues to enjoy running marathons, and has completed twenty-two marathons, including seven at Boston. Please e-mail her at dherring12@tampabay.rr.com.

Claire Howlett is an eighth grade student in Connecticut. She enjoys running, reading, and playing the piano. Claire would like to thank her siblings and parents for constantly supporting her.

Jeff Hoyt received a BFA from the University of Nevada, Las Vegas in 2004. He performs stand-up with a local comedy troupe and one day hopes to run with every Hash House Harrier kennel in the world. You can e-mail him at alcoholidayhhh@gmail.com.

Humorist and author **Roberta Beach Jacobson's** credits include *Chicken Soup for the Beach Lover's Soul* and *Chicken Soup for the Dieter's Soul*. She makes her home on a far-flung Greek island. Learn more by visiting her website: www.RobertaBeachJacobson.com.

Jennifer Lee Johnson is a writer and editor based in Baltimore, MD. She is currently working on her first novel. You can read more of her work at www.jen-johnson.com.

Rachel Jones is a freelance writer and international development worker. She lives in Djibouti with her family. She has been a contributing writer to *Running Times* magazine. Rachel has run on four continents and writes about running and daily life in Africa. E-mail her at trjones@securenym.net.

Ron Kaiser, Jr. lives and teaches English in New Hampshire, and has somehow managed to trick an almost disturbingly beautiful woman to marry him. He is quite satisfied with himself because of this. His other passion is writing fiction, and he is currently seeking representation for a collection of short stories and a novel. Contact him via e-mail at kilgore.trout1922@gmail.com.

Fallon Kane is sixteen years old and has wanted to be a writer since she was five. She loves reading, acting, fitness, and, of course, writing! Fallon lives with her mother and twin brother, who are pretty much the best mother and brother anybody could ask for.

Christina Kapp is a writer living in New Jersey with her husband and two daughters. She looks forward to her second and third triathlons in 2010 and is working on her first novel. She blogs at http://booksandcrayons.wordpress.com.

Machille Legoullon is a children's book author, wife, and proud mother of four boys. She is currently working on her first middle grade novel and has completed a picture book manuscript she is hoping to publish soon. Machille is extremely involved with her sons' school and the family business. E-mail her at writerinside@comcast.net.

Erin Liddell is a pseudonym for a writer living and ministering in south-central Pennsylvania.

Nancy Liedel is an amateur triathlete, mom of four special needs boys, writer and home educator. She also owns her own cosmetics company. Nancy loves to run, bike and deals with the swim section of a Tri. Winning, to Nancy, is just getting through the race.

Bobbie Jensen Lippman is a writer who lives with her husband Burt, their dog Charley and a shelter cat named "Lap Sitter." Bobbie's work has been published nationally and internationally. She writes a human interest column called "Bobbie's Beat" for the *Newport* (Oregon) *News-Times*. She is also a motivational speaker. She can be contacted at bobbisbeat@aol.com.

For the past eleven years, **Rita Lussier's** column entitled "For the Moment" has been a popular weekly feature in *The Providence Journal*. She lives with her husband, two children and their black Lab in Jamestown, RI. She can be reached via e-mail at ReetsAL@aol.com.

Dr. Tim Maggs has been a sports medicine chiropractor for thirty-one years and a sports medicine columnist for running magazines throughout the country. He is the developer of The Structural Management® Program, a sports biomechanics program. Dr. Maggs lives in upstate New York with his wife and four sons. E-mail him at RunningDr@aol.com.

Scott Maloney received his BS from Becker College in 2005. This is his second entry in the *Chicken Soup for the Soul* series. He enjoys traveling the country as a motivational speaker addressing audiences of all ages. Contact Scott via e-mail at info@scottmaloney.com or visit www.scottmaloney.com.

Dana Martin is a writer living in Bakersfield, California, with her husband of twenty-one years and their three children. Dana has a bachelor's degree in English and is the president of Writers of Kern (a branch of the California Writers Club). She enjoys camping, movies, and watching her son play professional baseball. E-mail her at DanaMartin14@gmail.com.

Carolyn Magner Mason is a freelance writer living in Tuscaloosa, AL. She teaches writing at The University of Alabama and writes for fitness, travel, regional and trucking publications. She enjoys running and traveling with her husband and two daughters. Please e-mail her at carolynmason76@yahoo.com.

Chuck Matsoff is a freelance writer and is currently working on a number of book projects. He is married to Angie and they have three sons, Austin, T and Blaze. Chuck enjoys running, cycling and riding his Harley as often as possible. Please e-mail him at cmatsoff52405@yahoo.com.

Bonnie Schey McClurg received her Bachelor of Arts from Moody

Bible Institute in 2001. She enjoys speaking and teaching on the Christian life and is a member of Writer's Bloc in Granbury, TX. She has six grandchildren and continues to swim, bike and run. E-mail her at bonniemcclurg@charter.net.

Amy Stockwell Mercer is a freelance writer living in Charleston, SC with her husband and three sons. She is running every day and still likes to think of "Dita" when she needs an extra push. Read more of her writing at www.alsmercer.wordpress.com.

Carrie Monroe lives and writes in Minneapolis, MN. She works at a theater and has had stories published in children's magazines. She enjoys writing, biking, swimming and running. Check out her blog at www.kiwislife.blogspot.com.

Amy Moritz is a sportswriter and triathlete in Buffalo, NY. A graduate of St. Bonaventure University and the University at Buffalo, she writes about her continued exploration of endurance sports competition on her website www.amymoritz.wordpress.com.

Marianne Mousigian earned her Bachelor of Science with High Distinction from the University of Michigan in 2009. She enjoys running marathons, cycling, swimming, and yoga. Marianne plans to integrate her passion for health and fitness with her kinesiology academic background to pursue a career in sports medicine. E-mail her at mmousigi@gmail.com.

Ben Mueller is an avid runner and triathlete who has competed in over 350 races from the 2-mile to the marathon distance. He currently teaches mathematics at Hinckley-Big Rock High School and Waubonsee Community College. He grew up in Sheboygan, WI and attended UW-Whitewater.

Sherrie Page Najarian is a freelance writer who lives in Richmond, VA.

She also edits an essay column for the Yale School of Nursing alumni magazine, *Yale Nursing Matters*. She is a YSN graduate, class of 1994.

Lindsay Nielsen is a psychotherapist and motivational speaker in Minneapolis, MN. She has been published in *Good Housekeeping* and *A Cup of Comfort for the Grieving Heart*. She is currently seeking a publisher for her memoir, *One Foot in Front of the Other*. Please contact her through her website www.lindsaynielsen.com.

Carla O'Brien has not attempted the sport of running. Her days are spent chasing a crawling baby and a toddler with sticky hands. She enjoys meeting new people and working as a hotel guest service agent. You will still find her, with the girls, cheering Dad on from the sidelines.

P.R. O'Leary spends his time writing and film-making in an effort to get out of his corporate cubicle job. In between these spurts of creativity he enjoys running, playing geeky board games, and collecting strange items. He lives in a geodesic dome in New Jersey. Learn more at his website www.proleary.com.

J.M. Penfold lives in Portland, OR. Please e-mail him at penfol35@yahoo.com.

Roy Pirrung is a world and American ultramarathon champion and record holder. Formerly a two-pack-a-day smoker and binge drinker, he was transformed through discovering his love of running. He wrote a weekly newspaper column and is currently a public speaker and writing his autobiography. Please e-mail him at ultraone@charter.net.

Connie K. Pombo is a freelance writer and inspirational speaker. She has published magazine articles and contributed to numerous anthologies, including *Chicken Soup for the Soul* and *A Cup of Comfort* books. She is the author of *Moms of Sons Devotions to Go* and *Trading Ashes for Roses*. Learn more at www.conniepombo.com.

When she isn't writing or editing, **Carol McAdoo Rehme** runs errands, runs after grandkids, runs the household—and might even run for office. Anything is possible! Coauthor of five gift books, she has compiled several others, most recently *Chicken Soup for the Soul: Empty Nesters*. Visit her at: www.rehme.com.

Lisa Levin Reichmann received her J.D. from Duke University School of Law in 1999. A former attorney, she is now raising her three children full-time in the Washington, DC Metro area. She is a certified running coach through the Road Runners Club of America (RRCA) and a competitive marathon runner and triathlete.

Mark Remy lives, writes, and runs in Pennsylvania's Lehigh Valley, where he is executive editor of RunnersWorld.com. He is the author of *The Runner's Rule Book: Everything a Runner Needs to Know—And Then Some* (Rodale, 2009) and the upcoming *The Runner's Field Manual—A Practical Guide to Practically Everything* (Rodale, 2010). Mark has run 18 marathons, with a personal best time of 2:46.

Scott Rigsby is the author of *UnThinkable: The True Story About the First Double-Amputee to Complete the World-Famous Hawaiian Ironman Triathlon* (Tyndale, 2008). He is also a sought-after public speaker who travels the country sharing his message about doing "the unthinkable." Visit him at www.scottrigsby.com. He thanks author Jenna Glatzer (www.jennaglatzer.com) for helping him share his story.

Tammy Ruggles lives in Kentucky and has written poetry, articles, short stories, and screenplays. Her first book, *Peace*, was published in 2005, and she has recently turned her attention to filmmaking.

Mike Sackett is a former marathon runner, retired writing teacher and the author of four novels, two children's books and many short stories, both fiction and non-fiction. His published works include "A Letter to My Sister" in *Chicken Soup for the Soul: The Cancer Book*. Contact Mike via e-mail at sackettmike4@gmail.com.

Chris Salstrom is a professional accountant and is currently working on her Master of Divinity. She has been a writer since childhood and has contributed to self-help publications and hopes to publish works of fiction in the future. Please e-mail her at salstroc@gmail.com.

Will Sanchez, a lifelong New Yorker, received his Masters in Mathematics from the Courant Institute and is a dedicated Chi Runner, having raised over $10,000 for charity through running and walking. He is a member of the Community Emergency Response Team (CERT) and Community Board #8, Manhattan. Contact him at gottarun.now@gmail.com.

Kathryn Schneeman has been a runner since age eleven, and is a former teacher and fashion model. She was a coordinator for the Archdiocese of St. Paul and Minneapolis in the Office for Marriage, Family and Life. She and husband, Eric, now have nine children—all athletes. The baby twins love the running stroller! E-mail her at kathyschneeman@aol.com.

Diane Shaw served eleven years as Executive Secretary to a Colorado Springs pastor; she now spends her time writing. Diane has been published in *Chicken Soup for the Soul* books and her church publication. Active in the writers' guild, Words for the Journey, you can visit her blog at http://needmorewordscs.blogspot.com.

Kathleen Shoop lives in Oakmont where she is a writer, mother, wife, and educator. Kathleen is lucky enough to manage those roles in some capacity each day. She has articles and essays published in local magazines and papers on a regular basis. Please send any correspondence to jakenmax2002@aol.com.

A believer in the power of adventure and wildness, **Eli Shostak** has crafted a life based on facilitating educational experiences in far-flung places. He lives in Mancos, CO, perched between the mountains and the deserts, where he has abundant opportunities to find inspiration running and writing. E-mail him at elishostak@gmail.com.

Allen Smith is an award-winning freelance writer living in Vail, CO. He writes about health, fitness and outdoor sports. Smith has a master's degree in exercise physiology and exercise specialist certification with the American College of Sports Medicine at San Diego State University.

Lisa Smith-Batchen's athletic achievements have appeared on the covers of *The New York Times*, *Los Angeles Times*, *The Washington Post* and *Winning Magazine*. She has appeared in *Runner's World*, *Sports Illustrated for Women*, *ESPN The Magazine*, *Outside* magazine, *UltraRunning*, *Trail Runner*, *Running Times* and numerous other national and international publications. Lisa has raised over 4.5 million dollars for orphans.

Amanda Southall is a freelance writer and graduate of Virginia Tech. She currently lives in Richmond, VA where she enjoys writing, running, hiking, and biking around town.

Mark Spangler is a former radio broadcaster who teaches students at Mankato West High School as a paraprofessional. His work has been published in *Lyrical Iowa*, *Esquire*, and other publications. He lives with his wife, son and dogs in Minnesota and is a graduate of Minnesota State University, Mankato.

Diane Stark is a former teacher turned freelance writer. She is the author of *Teachers' Devotions to Go*. She writes about the important things in life: her family and her faith. She lives in southern Indiana with her husband Eric and their five children.

Erika Tremper lives in Hillsborough, NJ, with her husband Chris and two twin daughters. She enjoys running, swimming, and reading. Please e-mail her at Erikatremper@comcast.net.

Sharon Van Zandt teaches fourth grade and loves reading and writing. She is currently working on her second middle grade novel. She is still jogging.

Katie Visco founded Pave Your Lane, a campaign designed to empower people to follow their passions. Promoting this message, in 2009, Katie ran solo across America, and became the second youngest and thirteenth woman to do so. Contact Katie at www.paveyourlane. com to learn about her future endeavors!

Bettie Wailes worked as a software engineer for nearly twenty-five years, until she started her own tutoring company. She has been running since 1978, and has completed numerous road races, including sixty-seven marathons. She is currently working on a memoir about her running experiences from the perspective of an older, slower runner.

Samantha Ducloux Waltz, an award-winning freelance writer in Portland, OR, currently has more than forty essays in the *Chicken Soup for the Soul* series, *A Cup of Comfort* series, and numerous other anthologies. She has also written fiction and nonfiction under the name Samellyn Wood. Learn more at www.pathsofthought.com.

Bonnie West is a Saint Paul, MN writer and yoga teacher who has published essays in *Woman's Day*, *Redbook* and *Ladies' Home Journal*. She has also been published in *Chicken Soup for the Shopper's Soul* and has a story about her dog Beasley in *The Ultimate Dog Lover* book. She has just completed a novel. Please e-mail her at yogabonnie@yahoo.com.

Marjorie Woodall lives in Nevada City, CA, where she works as a book editor and proofreader. You can reach her via e-mail at marjoriewoodall @hotmail.com.

Greg Woodburn is a twenty-year-old sophomore and Trustee Scholar at the University of Southern California where he runs on the track and cross country teams. Greg's nonprofit organization Share Our Soles (www.ShareOurSoles.org) collects, cleans, and then distributes new and used running and athletic shoes to disadvantaged youth. Contact him at Greg@ShareOurSoles.org.

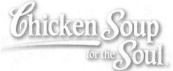

Meet Our Authors

Jack Canfield is the co-founder of Chicken Soup for the Soul and is also the co-author of many other bestselling books.

Jack is the CEO of the Canfield Training Group and founder of the Foundation for Self-Esteem. He has conducted intensive personal and professional development seminars on the principles of success for more than a million people in twenty-three countries, has spoken to hundreds of thousands of people, and has been seen by millions more on national television shows.

Jack has received many awards and honors, including three honorary doctorates and a Guinness World Records Certificate for having seven books from the *Chicken Soup for the Soul* series appearing on the New York Times bestseller list on May 24, 1998.

You can reach Jack at www.jackcanfield.com.

Mark Victor Hansen is the co-founder of Chicken Soup for the Soul. He is a sought-after keynote speaker and a prolific writer with many bestselling books in addition to the *Chicken Soup for the Soul* series. Mark has had a profound influence in the field of human potential through his library of audios, videos, and articles in the areas of big thinking, sales achievement, wealth building, publishing success, and personal and professional development. He is also the founder of the MEGA Seminar Series.

Mark has received numerous awards that honor his entrepreneurial spirit, philanthropic heart, and business acumen. He is a lifetime member of the Horatio Alger Association of Distinguished Americans.

You can reach Mark at www.markvictorhansen.com.

Amy Newmark is the publisher and editor-in-chief of *Chicken Soup for the Soul*, after a thirty-year career as a writer, speaker, financial analyst, and business executive in the worlds of finance and telecommunications. Amy is a *magna cum laude* graduate of Harvard College, where she majored in Portuguese, minored in French, and traveled extensively. She and her husband have four grown children, two of whom compete in the occasional triathlon.

After a long career writing books, financial reports, business plans, and corporate press releases, Chicken Soup for the Soul is a breath of fresh air for Amy. She has fallen in love with Chicken Soup for the Soul and its life-changing books, and really enjoys putting these books together for Chicken Soup's readers. She has co-authored more than two dozen *Chicken Soup for the Soul* books and has edited another two dozen.

You can reach Amy at webmaster@chickensoupforthesoul.com.

TIME magazine named **Dean Karnazes** one of the "Top 100 Most Influential People in the World," because he's expanded the limits of human endurance and, along the way, inspired others to be the best that they can be. His extraordinary endurance is legendary. *Wired* called him "The perfect human," and *Men's Fitness* says he "might just be the fittest man on the planet." For example, he's run 135 miles nonstop across Death Valley in 120-degree temperatures, and he's run a marathon to the South Pole in negative 40 degrees. He once ran 350 miles without rest.

Topping those feats, in 2006, he ran 50 marathons, in all 50 US states, in 50 consecutive days, finishing with the NY City Marathon, which he completed in three hours flat. In his free time, Dean is the *New York Times* bestselling author of *Ultramarathon Man: Confessions of an All-Night Runner* and *50/50: Secrets I Learned Running 50 Marathons in 50 Days—and How You Too Can Achieve Super Endurance!*, an entrepreneur, a philanthropist, and a devoted husband and father of two.

According to *The New York Times*, "Running with Karnazes is like setting up one' s easel next to Monet or Picasso." *Outside* called him "America's greatest runner." *The Philadelphia Inquirer* said of Dean, "He has not only pushed the envelope but blasted it to bits."

For more inspiration, visit Dean's website ultramarathonman.com.

Thank You!

"Dean dismisses boundaries. He makes everything seem possible," according to *The Washington Post*. It has been an honor to work with Dean Karnazes on this book, our very first volume ever for runners and triathletes. This superhuman man, who runs more miles in a week than most people run in their lives, is a regular hardworking guy—a husband, father, businessman, philanthropist, author and speaker, who also performs unbelievable feats of human endurance, inspiring hundreds of thousands of new runners along the way.

Dean collected stories from many of his friends, who are also pretty superhuman, and these are scattered throughout the book along with the stories from our regular high-performing contributors. We owe huge thanks to all of our contributors, not just the ones whose stories grace these pages. We can only publish a small percentage of the stories that are submitted, but we read every single one and even the ones that do not appear in the book have an influence on our thinking and on the final manuscript.

I want to thank Chicken Soup for the Soul editor Kristiana Glavin for reading the thousands of stories and poems that were submitted for this book. She helped us narrow down an incredibly high quality group of submissions. You runners are fit *and* smart, and you sure know how to write! I also want to thank D'ette Corona, our assistant publisher, who worked with all our contributors, and our editor and webmaster Barbara LoMonaco, for her expert proofreading assistance.

We owe a very special thanks to our creative director and book producer, Brian Taylor at Pneuma Books, for his brilliant vision for the high-impact cover and interior of this book. Finally, none of this would be possible without the business and creative leadership of our CEO, Bill Rouhana, and our president, Bob Jacobs.

~Amy Newmark
Publisher and Editor-in-Chief